T0264489

Group Work Stories Celebrating Diversity

Group Work Stories Celebrating Diversity is a most timely book about group work practice and education that highlights the theme of diversity, which encompasses acceptance and respect for various dimensions of difference. Dimensions of diversity include race, ethnicity, gender, sexual orientation, socio-economic status, age, physical or intellectual abilities, linguistic difference, religious beliefs, international or regional origin, lifestyle, political beliefs, or other ideologies, as well as the varying and complex intersection of these various dimensions. The thirty-one meaningful stories in this book explore these differences, leading to understanding and to moving beyond simple tolerance to mutual empathy, genuine and open encounter, and the celebration of the rich dimensions of diversity. Readers will enjoy this wonderfully intimate and intriguing collection, and will be moved to share them with others to help to spread the word about the importance of embracing, understanding and celebrating diversity. This book, with an international cast of authors – practitioners, educators and students – is a welcome antidote to the divisiveness and suspicion that swirl around difference and have become a sad hallmark of current times.

This book was originally published as a special issue of the journal *Social Work with Groups*.

Andrew Malekoff is Executive Director and CEO for North Shore Child and Family Guidance Center in Roslyn Heights, NY, USA, where he has worked since 1977. He has been editor of the quarterly professional journal *Social Work with Groups* since 1990, and is the author of *Group Work with Adolescents: Principles and Practice* (1997), now in its 3rd edition (2014).

Group Work Stories Celebrating Diversity

Edited by
Andrew Malekoff

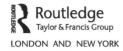
Routledge
Taylor & Francis Group

LONDON AND NEW YORK

First published 2018
by Routledge
2 Park Square, Milton Park, Abingdon, Oxon, OX14 4RN, UK

and by Routledge
711 Third Avenue, New York, NY 10017, USA

Routledge is an imprint of the Taylor & Francis Group, an informa business

Introduction, Chapters 1–16, 18–31 © 2018 Taylor & Francis
Chapter 17 © 2018 The Center for Harm Reduction Therapy

All rights reserved. No part of this book may be reprinted or reproduced or utilised in any form or by any electronic, mechanical, or other means, now known or hereafter invented, including photocopying and recording, or in any information storage or retrieval system, without permission in writing from the publishers.

Trademark notice: Product or corporate names may be trademarks or registered trademarks, and are used only for identification and explanation without intent to infringe.

British Library Cataloguing in Publication Data
A catalogue record for this book is available from the British Library

ISBN 13: 978-1-138-30241-9

Typeset in Minion
by RefineCatch Limited, Bungay, Suffolk

Publisher's Note
The publisher accepts responsibility for any inconsistencies that may have arisen during the conversion of this book from journal articles to book chapters, namely the possible inclusion of journal terminology.

Disclaimer
Every effort has been made to contact copyright holders for their permission to reprint material in this book. The publishers would be grateful to hear from any copyright holder who is not here acknowledged and will undertake to rectify any errors or omissions in future editions of this book.

Contents

CONTENTS

Citation Information

The chapters in this book were originally published in *Social Work with Groups*, volume 40, issues 1–2 (2017). When citing this material, please use the original page numbering for each article, as follows:

For any permission-related enquiries please visit:
http://www.tandfonline.com/page/help/permissions

Notes on Contributors

Samuel R. Benbow is Associate Professor in the Department of Social Work & Gerontology, Shippensburg University, PA, USA.

Jenilee Botha is a student at University of Pretoria, Pretoria, South Africa.

Jennifer A. Clements is Professor in the Department of Social Work & Gerontology, Shippensburg University, PA, USA.

Carol S. Cohen is Associate Professor at Adelphi University School of Social Work, NY, USA.

Edna W. Comer is Associate Professor in the School of Social Work, University of Connecticut, CT, USA.

Mark Doel is Emeritus Professor at the Centre for Health and Social Care Research, Sheffield Hallam University, UK.

Melissa Eaton is a Psychotherapist at the Center for Harm Reduction Therapy at Hospitality House, Sixth Street Self-Help Center, San Francisco, CA, USA.

Les Fleischer is Assistant Professor in the School of Social Work, Lakehead University, Canada.

Jan Fook is Professor of Higher Education Pedagogy at Leeds Trinity University, UK.

Maria A. Gurrola is Associate Professor in the School of Social Work, New Mexico State University, NM, USA.

Brandon Haydon is a Licensed Social Worker who has trained at Loyola University, Chicago, IL, USA.

Sarah R. Hemphill is a Licensed Social Worker who holds graduate degrees both in Social Work and Social Justice from Loyola University, Chicago, IL, USA.

Alexandria Holmes is the Data Enrollment Specialist at Denver Seminary, CO, USA.

Lee-Ann Human is a MSW (Health Care) student at the University of Pretoria, Pretoria, South Africa.

Carol Irizarry is Associate Professor in the School of Social and Policy Studies, Flinders University, Australia.

Narine N. Kerelian is a PhD candidate in the Department of Social Work and Social Administration, The University of Hong Kong.

Charlene Lane is Assistant Professor in the Department of Social Work & Gerontology, Shippensburg University, PA, USA.

Katrina Skewes McFerran is Professor of Music Therapy at the University of Melbourne, Australia.

Andrew Malekoff is Executive Director and CEO for North Shore Child and Family Guidance Center in Roslyn Heights, NY, USA.

Lindokuhle Maphalala is a BSW graduate from the University of Pretoria, Pretoria, South Africa.

Thato Masuku is a student at the University of Pretoria, Pretoria, South Africa.

Catherine K. Medina is Associate Professor in the School of Social Work, University of Connecticut, CT, USA.

Destinee Miguest has an MSW from Loyola University, Chicago, IL, USA.

Joshua L. Miller is Professor in the School for Social Work, Smith College, MA, USA.

Barbara Muskat is the Director of Social Work at the Hospital for Sick Children, Toronto, Canada.

Karen Myers is Assistant Professor in the Department of Social Work, James Madison University, VA, USA.

Lirio K. Negroni is Associate Professor in the School of Social Work, University of Connecticut, CT, USA.

Amy Nitza is Director of the SUNY New Paltz Institute for Disaster Mental Health, NY, USA.

Olufunke (Funke) Oba is a tenure-track faculty member at the University of Regina, Faculty of Social Work, Saskatoon, Saskatchewan, Canada.

Yuxin Pei is Associate Professor in the Department of Social Work and Sociology, Sun Yat-Sen University, Guangzhou, China.

Michael D. Pelts is Assistant Professor in the School of Social Work, University of Southern Mississippi, MI, USA.

Andrew J. Peters is Director of the Manhattan Center Program for the School of Social Work, Adelphi University, NY, USA.

Reineth Prinsloo is Associate Professor at the Department of Social Work and Criminology, University of Pretoria, Pretoria, South Africa.

Ann M. Rodio is Program Administrator with the Mississippi Department of Mental Health, USA.

Annie Pullen Sansfaçon is Associate Professor of Social Work, Université de Montréal, Canada.

Bharati Sethi is Assistant Professor at Kings School of Social Work, Western University, Canada.

Lawrence Shulman is the former Dean of SUNY Buffalo, NY, USA, where he was based in the School of Social Work.

Shirley R. Simon is Associate Professor in the School of Social Work, Loyola University, Chicago, IL, USA.

Rebecca L. Thomas is Associate Professor in the School of Social Work, University of Connecticut, CT, USA.

Michelle G. Thompson is a doctoral student in Social Welfare at Florida International University, FL, USA.

Zipho Tshapela is a BSW graduate from the University of Pretoria, Pretoria, South Africa.

George W. Turner is Associate Professor of Practice at the University of Kansas, KS, USA.

Evadné van den Berg is a student at University of Pretoria, Pretoria, South Africa.

Joseph Walsh is Professor of Social Work at Virginia Commonwealth University, VA, USA.

David Ward is Professor of Social and Community Studies at the School of Applied Social Sciences, De Montfort University, Leicester, UK.

Norissa J. Williams is Visiting Assistant Professor of Applied Psychology at New York University, USA.

Introduction

This special 40th Anniversary double-issue of *Social Work with Groups* was inspired by a conversation at the November 2014 board of directors meeting of the International Association for Social Work with Groups (IASWG). As a long-time board member, when the question was raised about what steps might be taken to advance the issue of diversity, I immediately thought that a special anniversary issue on the subject would be a step in the right direction.

Never one to let the grass grow under my feet, immediately after the board meeting I developed a rough draft of a "call for papers." I then asked a few of my fellow IASWG board members for their input. Following, in part, is the result of that collective effort:

> The *Social Work with Groups* journal, in concert with the International Association for Social Work with Groups, is inviting narrative essays of 5 to 10 manuscript pages, about group work practice that highlights the theme of diversity. Diversity encompasses acceptance and respect for various dimensions of difference. These can be along the lines of race, ethnicity, gender, sexual orientation, socio-economic status, age, physical or intellectual abilities, linguistic difference, religious beliefs, international or regional origin, political beliefs, or other ideologies and the varying and complex intersection of these various dimensions. The journal is seeking meaningful stories that explore these differences and that lead to understanding and moving beyond simple tolerance to mutual empathy, genuine and open encounter, and the celebration of the rich dimensions of diversity.
>
> A narrative essay is a story written about a personal experience. Writing a narrative essay provides an opportunity to get to know and understand oneself better and to shed light on an experience that may illuminate its meaning for others. One of the best ways to reveal who you are is to tell a story about how you became aware of something, gained a new way of seeing the world, a new insight. Your group work story should illustrate the interaction among group members and between group members and group workers in a way that brings the group encounter to life in a compelling way for readers. And, it should highlight what was learned from the experience that might be useful for readers who are practicing, teaching, or researching group work.

The "call for papers" went out soon thereafter and, as the July 1, 2015 deadline approached, stories started to trickle in. Brevity was encouraged and, so, I was concerned about receiving enough good manuscripts to complete one issue of the Journal. Despite my misgivings, more than enough stories arrived to fill a double issue!

As I started to read the stories I was captivated and moved beyond expectation. Many of the stories needed ongoing work to get the best out of them. I found that for some authors writing a manuscript that was not scholarly was a challenge. My number one suggestion to these authors was "less theory, more story." For me this evolved into an intimate process. I felt that I was getting to know the writers, some of whom were strangers to me, in a way that I never get to know writers who contribute to regular issues of the journal.

There was something about the storytelling process that enabled contributors to let down their guard and for me to ask questions that I had hoped would lead to deeper levels of revelation. For some authors, this seemed to come naturally. However, for most it required a "dialogue," that mostly happened through email correspondence.

After making final decisions on what to include, 31 stories in all, I had to decide how to organize the stories. Because there were more than I expected I wondered if I might group them into categories. And, although most stories are not mono-thematic, I did my best to classify them and give readers a range of general areas to choose from as they work their way through the collection.

I arrived at seven general themes: learning from the inside-out, growing up, aging, medical model to social model, language, in the classroom, and searching for meaning and more.

I hope that you will enjoy this wonderfully intimate and intriguing collection stories as much as I have and that you will share them with others to help to spread the word about the importance of embracing, understanding, and celebrating diversity. I don't need to explain to anyone reading this that in this world, at this time, we need to do that more than ever.

Many thanks to all of the authors for being so thoughtful, open and willing to put in the work to make sure that your stories were "just right."

Andrew Malekoff

FROM THE INSIDE-OUT

"When I let go of what I am, I become what I might be."

Lao Tzu

When the Trainer Got Trained: Seven Things I Learned About Delivering Diversity Trainings

Norissa J. Williams

Introduction

My diversity awakening

My introduction to ethnic diversity came earlier than most—particularly because the "otherness" of my family and I was evident, even in the smallest of things. My family had migrated to the United States from the twin Caribbean islands of Trinidad and Tobago. When they first moved to the country, they resided in a low-income, high-crime area in Brooklyn, New York. Following the American script, my family soon acquired enough collateral to move out of the city and to the suburbs in search of a better life.

My earliest schooling took place in Flatbush, Brooklyn—a place known then and now for its high concentration of Caribbean migrants. My pre-school teacher, with her sing-song accent, was reminiscent of my family—as she too had migrated from Trinidad. As such, when I learned to speak it was with the accent of those in my household, reinforced outside the home by this nursery school teacher. In this cultural enclave a growing child had no sense of "difference" to be aware of, as we all seemed the same. It wasn't until I had moved to Long Island, and attended schools where I was the only Trinidadian in sight, that I began to become aware of "difference." I remember most distinctly a time of guided learning in kindergarten as my teacher reviewed numbers with us. "One, two, tree—," I called out along with the rest of the class. Having heard me, my teacher Ms. Brant kindly stopped the class and gently corrected me, saying, "It's THR-ee (emphasizing the *TH* sound). TREE's grow outside." I remember being mildly shocked. After all, that's what I was taught at home, and that's how my nursery school teacher (and the entire class) said it! If I had had the courage I might have replied, "Um … I'm pretty sure it's TREE." However, being the shy, quiet, obedient child that I was, I adopted her pronunciation quickly. Days after this incident, in the kitchen of our home, my grandfather reviewed numbers with us again. He said, "One, two, tree—," and like Ms. Brant I quickly interrupted him and said, "No, it's THR-ee (emphasizing the *TH* sound). TREE's grow outside."

My grandfather's reply left me in a state of puzzlement again as I had already reconciled this issue in my head. I was clearly wrong and Ms. Brant was clearly right, I had thought, but here I was being told that I was wrong again. "It's TREE," he said, "We are from Trinidad."

The transformation that comes with an awakened perspective

Volumes were spoken in the few words my grandfather said. For one, I had come to the realization that though Ms. Brant and my family spoke English, they were speaking with different accents. One wasn't right, while the other wrong—just different. And though I didn't have the words to articulate as much, this incident was the start of my learning that my culture was something to be proud of and hold onto—not something I could let be easily invalidated. A lot more began to make sense to me about my family and the outside world, as well. I had an awakened understanding of diversity that would later shape my learning interests and career pursuits.

Although I feel fortunate to have ties in two countries it hasn't come without its challenges. Often faced with feeling, "other," because of my ethnicity, my race, my socioeconomic status, and more recently, my status as a divorced, single mother in Academia—I've been able to look at America's institutions with a critical eye, seeing opportunities for growth as it pertains to inclusion and diversity. As you might imagine, part of my lived experience has been associated with feelings of alienation and exclusion—from the racial stratification caused by educational tracking, leaving me one of few minorities in advanced classes, to sitting in graduate courses where the rare mention of Black people often came from a deficit perspective (i.e. "poverty," "at risk." etc.). Yet these experiences of being "other" have arguably become one of my greatest assets—infusing me with a love for diversity and leading me down paths of studying abroad, studies of cross-cultural differences and professional work in the field of cultural competence.

My work as the director of cultural and linguistic competence

Very early in my career, after receiving my masters in social work, still conscious of cross-cultural differences, I became concerned with cultural bias that existed in policies, laws, and the social services provided to racial and ethnic minorities. I thought critically of my family and Western conceptions of mental health and well-being and American ideals of family functioning. I saw how immediately my family would have been at a disadvantage had they had the misfortune of coming to the attention of Family Court—not because they were actually deficient, but because of the differences that existed between their cultural norms and those of American institutions. As such, when I returned to school to work on my doctoral degree, my research centered on cross-cultural differences in coping skills, help seeking, and other mental health–related behaviors. This naturally led to research in the area of cultural competence, as I believe, true cultural competence to be an answer to the bias that exists in policies and services. During my educational training I was fortunate enough to get an internship that parlayed into a paid position as a director of Cultural and Linguistic Competence. In this position I did a number of things to infuse principles of cultural and linguistic competence throughout the county in which I worked. The most significant of these things were the diversity trainings that I offered free of charge to local agencies.

These diversity trainings are the subject of the remainder of this article. The background provided heretofore set the backdrop upon which one can understand that I approached this work with a valuable amount of life experience and a solid practice and research background. Nonetheless, this work and participants in my trainings further transformed me and my understanding of and appreciation for diversity. In the next section, this article discusses insights I gathered while doing this work.

Lessons learned in the field

Lecture is Important but real change happens with empathy

Coming from a research and academic setting my inclination is to teach traditionally. So as I prepared for my first training, I asked myself normal teaching questions such as, "What are my main points? Have I supported it with enough research? Are my ideas clearly outlined on the PowerPoint?" and "Do I have some kind of handout that participants can go home with?" Although these questions are important and valid considerations, after doing my first three trainings and learning that most social work organizations are not equipped with the technical apparatus to allow my PowerPoint presentations, I focused on the questions and activities that I had included in my slides to drive home the main points. I quickly learned that people didn't remember the facts I taught them, and when they did, they often didn't remember them accurately, but what stayed with them was what they "felt." As such when I asked them to do activities such as role-plays, case vignettes, or an experience walk, I would ask them to focus on how they feel. Most of the time I would challenge them to think of minority groups they belong to— as we all belong to at least one or two. I would go so far as finding someone in the audience who was left-handed living in a right-handed world. With having someone from an oppressed group (that is not emotionally charged and socially loaded) discuss their experience I could then gently ascend with an unarmed group into more negatively charged, socially loaded discussions, such as race. I would assist and give language to the things they experienced and make connections that they might not have otherwise seen. Although you can never win them all, with this approach I often received very good verbal and written feedback as their eyes were opened.

Decreasing social distance and increasing contact between participants will change lives

Over time I have learned that the best way to create a learning environment in the context of diversity is to help people see that we are more alike than we are different. This goes along with my first point that discusses the importance of fostering empathy in your participants. In fact, this point may be the flip side of empathy. One activity that I adopted after being a participant in an excellent training was "Concentric Conversations." In this activity I choose about four or five questions related to the topic of the training and I have people pair up with partners to discuss these things. One of the first directives I typically give is, "Talk about where you grew up and share a fond memory from there." This usually opens the floor and disarms people, making the following questions easier. Thereafter, depending on what the overall topic of my training is, I can say something else like, "Talk about the time you first witnessed or experienced an ism." With these questions, even in settings where participants have worked together for years, and it would be assumed that they knew one another, inevitably participants learn something brand new about people whose desks were right next to theirs. Ultimately you learn, "You can't judge a book by its cover." You have to take time to engage deeply with people to experience your shared humanity.

Once there was a petite, very conservatively dressed young White woman who stated that she was a punk-rocker by weekend and psychiatrist by weekday. One would never know from mere observation that she was into the punk lifestyle. Another time, two seemingly racially and ethnically different people realized, though they lived far from where they started life, they originated from the same place. Once people begin to experience similarities and the lines are blurred between, "us" and "them," social distance is decreased. The floor is set for empathy for the others experience. A sense of shared humanity takes the floor and people get protective of one another—passionate about each other's causes.

You can disarm your audience by sharing your own shortcomings

The most challenging of topics that I, a Black woman, could approach in a county where service providers were predominantly White, was ... (you guessed it) race! As such, because I had previously worked in the county and lived in neighboring counties, I was well aware that I had to approach the issue wisely. Initially, nervous that I would be perceived as the "angry

Black woman," or be thought to be using "the race card," I gave a lot of thought to my approach. In some settings, even though this was what I had been hired for, I could not outright approach the topic of race. I was however safe discussing the more socially acceptable topic of "diversity," without giving the oppression I was discussing a race. People were more comfortable that way. To go further with these audiences, as a tool, I used self-disclosure to disarm participants. I told stories of my shortcomings and unfair biases that I may have had. In so doing I not only humanized myself, and took away this feeling of finger pointing, I joined them by admitting to work that I also had to do. These light-hearted, humorous stories also stirred memories and helped them to identify their own unintended biases. The environment felt safer to participants. They could risk exposure, because I had.

Be sure to know who you are training

I once made the mistake of assuming that all audiences in this county were pretty much the same. As such even though I was going to an audience that was not composed of my typical seasoned social work crowd, I approached them with my usual joviality. I introduced myself, my professional role and stated that I was also a doctoral student. Within minutes I was accused of being racist (though I had not even had the opportunity to discuss race), and was insulted by an audience member who insinuated that the only reason I got into a doctoral program was affirmative action, "Which is really such a shame, seeing as how perfectly good White people were probably passed up." It took everything in me to gather myself in front of this audience—especially because the training had not even begun. It was a tough session to get through as defenses were up. Fortunately, I later had the opportunity to go back better prepared. Nonetheless I learned a valuable lesson. Education, prior exposure, current professional roles, the context of diversity fostered within the work environment, and other important factors, were important things to consider when contracted to do work for an agency. Learning will not take place without tailoring your message to the unique culture of those you are serving.

Everyone has a meaningful story to share. Encourage them to share it

As with any audience, there will be varying degrees with which people feel comfortable sharing things publicly. However, most learning occurs from the people in the audience as opposed to from just the trainer themselves. The trainer must be skilled in drawing stories out, weaving stories together, and drawing collective meaning from participants lived experiences. One of the most meaningful experiences I had when delivering training came when a woman who identified herself as a lesbian in a same-sex relationship shared what it took for her and her partner to schedule vacations. As a heterosexual woman I don't have to consider looking for vacation spots where I could hold hands with my partner publicly. I could find a man I met two minutes ago and hold hands or kiss in public (I wouldn't of course), and may not be looked at twice. I was afforded a luxury by virtue of heterosexual privilege that she was not. Although not exact, that experience of marginalization was something that I could relate to. My prior experiences of oppression enabled me to deeply feel what she had experienced. In fact, I sat with that in our group session and we all felt it. We had been together for three 8-hour sessions and had developed a camaraderie that caused us to become allies for each other. We shared many stories like that. One woman discussed what it was like to be Chinese in an American context, whereas another shared what it was like to be poor and Jewish in a middle-class, White neighborhood. Another man shared the disrespect he endured as a doctor with a heavy foreign accent. Members empathized with the pain of the others. Bonds were formed, and conceptual bridges were crossed.

Do not ignore intersections of Identity

The existence of oppression, inequity, and unfairness that exists for some groups, as compared to others, necessitates the promotion of diversity. In fact, in many ways, the embracing and celebration of diversity can serve as one part of an antidote to oppression. However, when we talk about oppression, we think if it as it pertains to race, class, gender, sexuality, and so on. In my earlier trainings, and I still find myself falling into this trap every now and again, I would speak about one form of oppression or another—as though they were unilaterally experienced. However, this couldn't be further from the truth. There are those that experience multiple layers of oppression. The poor, transgender, Black man has a very different experience than an upper-class, transgender, White man by virtue of the ways these multiple identities intersect. This intersectionality needs to be addressed when discussing oppression and diversity. Not only does it give an observer a lens through which one can more accurately view oppression, it also validates the lived experience of those whose multiple identities intersect to complicate the existence of any one form of oppression. Furthermore, acknowledging and including education of these things in one's discussion gives a language to those who are oppressed and those who seek to be allies to address oppression.

Use people's discomfort for learning

As earlier stated, my personality, especially in group settings, is more shy and quiet. I prefer to get along with people. As such, I don't like confrontations and would shy away from them. This means when I first started doing these trainings and uncomfortable things would occur, such as people rolling their eyes, folding their arms, or walking out of the room, I would try to ignore it—though it bothered me well beyond the end of the training. Eventually I got comfortable enough to use these things in my training sessions. Often I'd normalize the experience of discomfort. "The things we're talking about today are uncomfortable. However, this is a safe environment to discuss this discomfort. If you left here with unprocessed discomfort or anger, then I haven't really done my job." I may then look directly at someone and say, "I've noticed that you've shifted in your seat, rolled your eyes, huffed and whispered to your partner a few times in the last 10 minutes. Would you feel comfortable sharing what you're feeling?" More often than not people become aware of their behavior. There have been a few times when people minimize it and attribute it to something else. However, the majority of times people get really nice (because they don't want to seem like the bad guy/gal) and share their discomfort politely. Most times, before I could address what was expressed, another participant would jump in and offer something they learned whether in the training session or prior to, to help them when they've felt similar ways. If participants don't volunteer, I may open it up to the crowd and ask them their thoughts on the matter. This has proven to be a very useful strategy in my training practice time and time again.

Conclusion

I began this piece taking you on a journey through my early life, highlighting my first experience of being "other" and my embrace of diversity. I then shared with you how these things affected my educational and career choices—infusing this journey of mine, with nothing short of richness and life. Thereafter, I shared with the reader the many lessons I learned from participants when delivering diversity trainings. However, what I'm about to conclude with may be the most important part of this article, as it is the ultimate summation of all that I have learned through personal experience, education and the professional practice of promoting diversity. The lesson is simple, cultural competence, harmony and diversity boils down to love and mutual respect. That almost sounds too simple to be profound. However, its profoundness is better experienced than discussed. Suffice it to say, in whatever diversity work one does, they should seek to create a feel good atmosphere that is safe for the disclosure of uncomfortable confessions of and questions about individual biases. When one can do that, one can plant a seed or even completely transform the ways in which people embrace difference.

Addressing Internalized Biases and Stereotypes of the Group Leader: A Life-Long Professional Task

Lawrence Shulman

It doesn't matter how long you have been in the field, how much professional work you have done on issues of diversity, how sensitive you may be to avoid microaggressions when dealing with differences, or how committed you are to your professional association's code of ethics, your early internalized biases and stereotypes may sometimes emerge. When this happens, it's a reminder that it can take a lifetime of professional work to fully understand all of what you unconsciously believe and feel, and the many ways these thoughts and feelings can sneak up on you. This issue of the *Journal* provides an opportunity to share a number of personally embarrassing experiences, each one having taught me not only more about myself as a person and as a professional, but also how to work more effectively with groups on certain taboo issues.

I start by explaining that I am somewhat versed in the literature on intercultural (e.g., White social worker dealing with an African American client) and intracultural (e.g., a Hispanic social worker dealing with a Hispanic client) issues. I have published on this subject (Shulman, 2002, 2005, 2016), produced videotape programs coled with an African American female colleague (Clay & Shulman, 1994), taught about the subject to MSW and PhD students and conducted numerous training workshops for social workers, supervisors and administrators. That's in part what made these incidents embarrassing from my perspective; however, they were also enlightening. I am a White, Jewish, straight male, born and raised in an essentially White, working-class neighborhood in Brooklyn, New York; all factors that I believe are relevant to the incidents described below.

A microaggression dealing with race

The first example occurred when I was teaching at the Boston University School of Social Work (BUSSW). I was presenting a continuing education 2-day (Friday—Saturday) workshop on inter- and intracultural issues in practice. The room was packed with 100 participants.

We had a reasonably good start on this sensitive topic on Friday with participants sharing examples after I discussed contracting with the group and threw out some "handles for work"—examples that had been raised at previous workshops. I also led the group in an exercise by asking participants to think about what made it hard to talk about such taboo subjects as race, gender, sexual orientation, and so on, and what would make it easier. As frequently happens, participants began to discuss how difficult these discussion can be. For example a White worker said, "I'm walking on egg shells because I'm afraid I will say the wrong thing or use the wrong word and then be attacked by the group." I acknowledged that she and others may have taken a course on oppression during their professional training that they had experienced as oppressive. Many in the workshop agreed. This opened up other examples by White participants of experiences dealing with gender, race, sexual orientation, and so on, that had resulted in their opting to stay quiet, not say anything in a workshop, a class, or at their agency. In this way, they avoided making a "mistake."

I pointed out we had not heard from any African American participants, or others who experience minority status, on what made it hard and what would make it easier to get into these difficult areas. One African American worker shared how she feels when White workers at agency staff meetings at which she is in the minority turn to her and say, "And what do your people think?" Her reaction is anger because she does not believe she is a spokesperson for "her people," and in addition, there is a lot of diversity within diversity. African Americans may think differently about things. Another Black participant said, "I get angry when I'm asked to 'educate' my white colleagues. They should care enough about this issue to do some research on their own." A young, male African American child welfare worker described a home visit with a White family investigating a report of neglect. During the visit the wife/mother referred to him as "sir." This was followed quickly by the husband saying, "You don't have to call him sir." The worker was understandably upset but said nothing. When I asked him what his supervisor had to say about that interview, he said, "Nothing, because I didn't tell her about that part." When I asked why, he replied "Well, she is White." They had never discussed their own intercultural difference, and thus he didn't feel comfortable sharing that with her.

Note that when workshop participants discuss how hard it is to talk about "it," they are actually talking about "it." The very discussion about the difficulties in addressing taboo subjects is actually starting to alter the norm of the workshop group's culture. When I asked what would make it easier, right here in the current workshop, suggestions included allowing people to risk and make mistakes without jumping on them with accusations of racism, sexism or homophobia. One African American member in the workshop added, "I wouldn't mind sharing my views on how my Black clients experience white workers and their agencies if I thought people really wanted to hear."

Following this conversation, participants put forward a number of inter- and intracultural examples for discussion and analysis over the 2-day workshop. I made a practice presentation to set the stage followed by discussion of their specific examples touching on gender, race, ethnicity, and sexual orientation. My sense was the day had gone well for a first day, recognizing that we might get into even more difficult and risky areas during the second day; however, the room was too warm and the thermostat was locked. The day ended with no response to my repeated calls to building maintenance to please adjust the thermostat.

Most people arrived on Saturday in casual clothing and the session began on time at 9:00AM. At about 9:20 I noticed a young African American male (not the one who had raised the issue the day before), in jeans, a sweat shirt, and baseball cap entering the back of the packed room. He looked around the room, and I said, "Thank you for coming. The thermostat is over there," pointing toward the wall. He paused and then said he was not the maintenance man, he was a participant and he was sorry he was late. I immediately felt embarrassed and apologized to him. He found the empty seat he had been searching for.

From that point on I was sweating but tried to continue my presentation. I noticed four African American women sitting in the first row looking at each other, whispering and nodding. After 5 minutes I knew I couldn't just continue on and acknowledged how upset I was about what I had just said. I continued:

> Here I am leading a workshop on intercultural issues and I didn't recognize John and assumed he was the maintenance man. This is a classic example of a micro-aggression and I am terrible sorry for that. I guess it tells me and all of us how easy it is to respond in that way.

All four of the African American women in the first row smiled and nodded, and one said, "We were wondering how long it would take for you to stop and really acknowledge what just happened. Not bad, since it only took about 5 minutes." I could sense an immediate lowering of tension in the room. John said, "It's OK, I'm use to that." I replied, "It was not OK. I guess it tells me that as hard as we try there is an underlying, gut stereotyping that takes place and should not happen." The reaction in the room was dramatic as participants, Black and White, straight and gay, started to share difficult incidents they had experienced with staff and clients and embarrassing mistakes of their own. A number of workers who were gay, who had not revealed their sexual orientation at their agencies, added their painful moments when straight staff made homophobic comments at meetings not realizing they were gay. It was clear that my honest acceptance of the inherent racism in my mistake, and my willingness to acknowledge it, unlocked the group participants' restraint and opened up the work. It also, in retrospect, modeled what they needed to do with clients when they made similar mistakes. Another example of how "more is caught than taught."

Internalized homophobia emerges while meeting with AIDS action staff

A second example, which also took place while I was on faculty at BUSSW occurred during a summer when I volunteered to present a workshop on group work at the downtown Boston office of the AIDS Action Committee. This was earlier in the epidemic when AIDS was characterized as a disease mostly affecting males who were gay and White. Preparing for the workshop, I used the skill of "tuning in." How would this group react to a straight, social work faculty member leading a session to offer them advice on their group practice? Although I had recently led a year-long group for persons with AIDS in early substance abuse recovery in a residence run by the agency, participants were not aware of that experience.

I also tuned in to my own feelings, remembering growing up in Brooklyn as a teenager who would go along with other teens my age when they made disparaging homophobic remarks and jokes. I reflected on the fact that my neighborhood in Williamsburg had, at that time, a large Chasidic (ultra-orthodox) community whose male members wore dark clothing, fur-lined hats, and had side locks of hair (Pe'ot) curing down their cheeks When a member of that group passed by and one of my peer group would make an anti-Semitic comment to a Chasid, I would stay silent. I remember feeling embarrassed, but I was embarrassed by the recipient of the anti-Semitism, and not by my peer making the comment. After all, I was Jewish as well, but not like them. I was different; they (the Chasid's) were the outsiders.

Feeling well tuned in to my own feelings and anticipating those of the AIDS Action staff, I arrived at the building and entered the elevator. I was accompanied by two tall construction men with muscle shirts, hard hats, and tool belts. I had never been to the AIDS Action office before. When the elevator door opened on the fourth floor reception area a large sign said, "AIDS Action Center." I immediately felt as if I wanted to turn to the construction men and say, "I'm straight." I didn't say it, but I felt like saying it. Where did that feeling come from? Also, why did I assume those men were straight?

When I walked into the conference room, I was faced by a group of about 30 staff members seated around a table. Most had their arms folded across their chests in the classic, nonverbal group signal of "go ahead, try to tell me something." I began as follows, "A funny thing just happened to me while riding up the elevator" and then described the experience and my immediate emotional reaction. As I did this, I could see the arms coming down and smiles on the faces of the participants. My acknowledging the homophobic reaction, once again, as with the intercultural workshop presentation, was crucial in setting a good tone for the 2-hour presentation. For the staff members who were gay, my recognition of this reaction, its meaning, and my willingness to share the incident, helped to overcome our intercultural differences.

What I also found interesting is that about 25% of the staff members around the table were straight. They shared that they had never discussed with their colleagues at this agency some of the issues they faced with friends, families, and other professionals when they disclosed that they worked at AIDS Action. With the ice melting, the group norm was modified to encourage discussion of this taboo topic. The workshop focused effectively on the inter- and intracultural issues faced by workers who are straight and who are gay as they interacted with their clients.

What do I make of these experiences?

Learning about ourselves, who we really are, never stops, nor should it. Pretending that because we have gone to a school of social work we have changed, and that all of the life experiences that shaped us no longer have a subconscious impact is naïve and delusional. We may have developed a sense of fairness toward others, and an understanding of the powerful impact sexism, racism, homophobia, social classism, privilege, attitudes toward the mentally and physically challenged, ageism, and so on has on all of us. We may have rejected these prejudices in our society. We may even have worked to fight these stereotypes and prejudices through social action in our agencies, community, and the political system; however, I believe there remain within all of us elements of our early family and community conditioning.

Those of us who are social work educators and supervisors have a responsibility to guard against communicating a vision of social workers as unbiased professionals, who constantly live and breathe the National Association of Social Workers Code of Ethics. Instead, we must create the conditions where those we educate and supervise feel free to explore even the most taboo thoughts and feelings, and to help them understand that this is a life-long personal and professional task. We should make clear that we will all make mistakes, learn from them, and then make more sophisticated mistakes. We can model this process by being honest about ourselves as I tried to be in the two examples above.

Writing this brief article reminded me of an incident in a practice class I taught in an MSW graduate program. It was the first class of the semester and a first class for most of the students. As we were discussing someone's case example, what I call problem swapping, a young White male made the comment, "That's the problem with these people" referring to an inner-city, African American client.

When he said that, I could see the looks on the faces of the other students responding to his "these people" description of the clients.

This is a crucial moment in a class because I could have responded by criticizing his comment and letting him know that this kind of language and attitude was not acceptable in social work. If I did, I would silence him, and perhaps others in the class, who would not risk making a similar mistake. Instead, I said I had noticed a number of students in the class reacting to his use of the term *these people*, as I had as well. I then told him that though I disagreed with his comment, I thought it took some courage in his first practice class, to share a comment like that. I then asked why he had used that phrase. This led to his describing for the class his growing up in "Southie," a mostly White working-class area of Boston that had erupted when bussing was introduced to integrate the schools. Also, his family had expressed negative views about Blacks. He was hearing it from family members and friends questioning why he was going to be a social worker and work with "these people."

This opened up a discussion for the entire class about reactions from friends and family members when they said they were studying at a school of social work. They were able then to share some of their own doubts and inherent biases. One young woman described coming from a middle-class, White suburb and never having had significant contacts in her community or school with persons of color. Another shared the biased comments she had heard from her family members and friends. When she tried to challenge them it always resulted in an escalation of the conflict.

The moral of the story and of this article is that we must work to be less harsh in judging ourselves, who we are and how we got to where we are. My comment to the young man in the class I just described was the start of my trying to change the culture of the group so that students didn't say what they thought the instructor and their peers wanted to hear, but rather what they really thought and felt. A student making a comment like this in the first class, in my view, is really saying to the school, albeit very indirectly, "Will you help me figure out if I belong here?" He was the "deviant member" raising an issue often felt by others in the group. If the same comment is made by the student in the 2nd year, then the responsibility of faculty and supervisors is to serve as gatekeepers and make sure this still-biased student does not graduate. In the meantime, I (and the reader) need to continue to learn who we are, what our buried prejudices may be, and how to overcome them in order to practice and teach in an ethical manner.

References

Clay, C., & Shulman, L. (1994). *Teaching about practice and diversity: Content and process in the classroom and the field.*(A series of eight videotaped programs co-produced with Cassandra Clay and distributed by the Council on Social Work Education, www.cswe.org).

Council on Social Work Education (Producer). (1993). *Teaching about practice and diversity: Content and process in the classroom and the field* [Video]. Alexandria, VA: Council on Social Work Education.

Shulman, L. (2002). Learning to talk about taboo subjects: A life long professional task. In R. Kurland & A. Malekoff (Eds.), *Stories celebrating group work: It's not always easy to sit on your mouth.* New York, NY: Haworth Press.

Shulman, L., with A. Gitterman (2005). *Mutual aid groups, vulnerable & resilient populations and the life cycle* (3rd ed.). New York, NY: Columbia University Press.

Shulman, L. (2016). *The skills of helping individuals, family, groups and communities* (8th ed.). Monterey, CA: Brooks/Cole, Cengage Publishers.

Invisible People Don't Need Masks

Jennifer A. Clements

The group that I cofacilitate is a weekly teen boys group in a somewhat urban area just 50 miles outside of Baltimore, Maryland. The boys who are in the group attend the meetings because they have lost a loved one recently and have been identified by their school counselor as having "behavioral difficulties." From a purely diagnostic perspective, these boys are diagnosed with oppositional defiant disorders, attention-deficit disorder, and depression. They come from homes where their parents are in jail, deceased, or unavailable. This is our 3rd month together, so I know more than what was on the initial assessment.

The boys are leaders, comedians, and poets. They have artistic spirits that make our art therapy group very special. They shared that they wanted to make a difference in the world when they grow up. Very early on the boys had decided to name the group the Difference Makers. They choose this name because they would be making things every week and said that the work they are doing might make a difference—thus, ***Difference Makers.***

We began the group with our usual check-ins. The kids were anxious to find out what we are making today in our group. The boys were unusually quiet and sharing in a very limited way. When we said that we would be making masks today, one of the boys mumbled under his breath but loud enough to hear, "Masks for kids who are invisible, great." I had heard it but was not sure who else had. I felt a mixture of anxiety and concern. I decided to reach out to him. "What was that Sam?" He quickly shut down and said, "Nah, sorry Ms. Jen. It's nothing." But it was something. I knew it and he knew it, as it just lingered in the air.

I will give some context to this group that will help you to understand where we are at this moment of awkward silence. It is April 2015 and a short drive outside of our little group is a city on fire. As Baltimore was planning the funeral of Freddie Gray, the city exploded. There are videos shown of people expressing violence and rage throughout Baltimore less than 3 weeks after this 25-year-old man died in police custody.

On April 12, 2015, Freddie Gray, a 25-year-old African-American man, was arrested by the Baltimore (Maryland) Police Department, reportedly for possessing an illegal switchblade. Although Gray was being transported in a police van, he fell into a coma. He was then taken to a trauma center. He died on April 19, 2015. His death has been attributed to injuries to his spinal cord that some believe occurred during the police transport due to his not being properly secured. Others believe his injuries were the result of the use of unnecessary force by the police. Six Baltimore police officers were temporarily suspended with pay, awaiting an investigation of the incident.

It is all over the media, and you cannot avoid it. It is not the city we know and love, yet it is the city we know in so many other ways. I know these kids on the streets, the ones the media is calling thugs and yet I don't know them. I can't really know them or their story because I am not Black. I am a White social worker reeking of privilege that the boys in my group will likely never know. I am generally aware of this in group, but I am especially aware of this difference today.

The comment that Sam made under his breath is sitting in my head. I look over at my cofacilitator as she hands out materials. She is smiling and moving forward without the knowledge I have that there is unrest here in the group. I am storing the comment away for now with the hope that the activity will allow for sharing. I do this, in part, because I think the painting will allow for a level of discussion that can be very intimate. During painting eyes are off of each other and talk on top of the activity might happen. I'm also afraid. I am afraid of where the discussion will go and fearful that it will not be productive. I am afraid that because I am different and cannot possibly relate to them, that I cannot help them to be heard and that they will experience me as one more person who will reject them—the "kids who are invisible," as Sam murmured a few minutes ago. I am afraid.

The session moves forward and we explain to the boys what they will be making today. The goal of the session is to make masks with images on the front of the mask that show how you present yourself to the world and images on the inside of the mask that depict only what you know.

It is a risk-taking activity and we are hoping the boys will share and express their vulnerability, as the tone has already been set in the previous groups. But today I have some doubts about if it is fair to ask them to do this with so much unrest in the air.

Paints are being passed around, and each boy has a blank mask to start with. Some of them jump right in, and some of them look like they are lost. Our goal as group workers is to silently support each member as he works on his art. The boys who struggle right now might be planning or thinking through ideas. I walk around the outside of the circle and check in with each one. After a few minutes they are all at work—painting and creating their masks. Some of the boys talk and share as they work and others work in silence. When everyone feels like they are finished, we begin the work of sharing.

James speaks up first, as is typical for the group. He says that the outside of his mask is painted "all Black because that is how everyone sees me all the time," and the inside of his mask is his version of the flag for France. He says that he wants to be a chef and that he hasn't told that to anyone except for his aunt. The boys are supportive as he shares and also tease him a bit as is their usual style.

I ask the group the question, "Let's compare the inside of the mask with the outside, what do you all think?" One of the boys states that the masks cannot exist together. He clarifies by saying, "You are not ever going to find a Frenchie Chef who's Black, ain't no way that is happening." I ask the rest of the group if they think that is true. Sam, the boy who made the comment at the beginning of the group speaks up, "It's not on being Black, it's invisible. Nobody sees you. That's why you gotta set things on fire, just to be seen." I try to imagine that, imagine that to be seen or heard in the world that I would have to set something on fire. I cannot imagine it.

The boys all seem to jump in to the conversation, as if permission had been granted for them to talk about Baltimore. They begin to share stories of large and microaggressions that they have experienced. The stories are hard to hear but not surprising.

My cofacilitator states that this is the first time we have ever talked about racism. She wonders out loud why that might be the case. The kids chime in, in resounding agreement that they did not want to make us feel bad. I roll that statement around in my head—did not want to make the facilitators, the people in the room charged with helping them, feel bad! I have a sickening feeling in the pit of my stomach that I have failed them.

For months we have been working along and have failed to address the elephant in the room. They feel invisible, and we have not even acknowledged that! The only thing I can think of to come out of my mouth is that I'm sorry.

"Well I want to say to you all that I am sorry. I am sorry that I did not bring this up and I am sorry that you feel like you need to spare my feelings." I share with them how it is hard for me to understand that boys with so much life in them could ever feel invisible but that for the first time today, I am beginning to understand. Another boy says that it is not just being invisible; it's that when people actually see him, they are afraid. He reports that "when I walk in town and a lady with her kid sees me and walks the other way 'cause she's scared of me, that hurts and it's not invisible. It's like De-Visible, something less or worse."

The boys agree with the idea of De-Visible, and we write that on a big sheet of paper. I ask them, "How do we work on this and how do we overcome it?" The boys write words all around the word that they think could counter it. The statements are interesting, expected things like "speak up" but also unexpected things like "sharing a sandwich." We have a good laugh about the sandwich and all agree that it is hard to be mad at someone when they are sharing their meal with you.

We are quickly running out of time. We do our wrap-up of what we got this week from group in one word each. *Real, truth,* and *honesty* are the words that are shared. We thanked them for taking the risk and hoped they would not worry about our feelings in group anymore. We want them to be themselves. The boys agree, some with smiles on their faces and some with tears in their eyes. The kids pile out of the room to leave group for the day. I say goodbye to each of them. As Sam leaves the room last, I say "goodbye Sam, you know that I see you right?" as tears well up in my eyes. Sam smiles back at me and says, "I know that you do now Ms. Jen."

"Small" Acts Are Often Not That Small

Mark Doel

I am a social group worker in northern England. For 20 years I worked in community-based settings (we called it "patchwork," better known outside the United Kingdom as "neighborhood work") and I practiced social work with groups, families, and individuals. Whilst I was a practitioner I started teaching social work at bachelors and masters levels and also leading training workshops for qualified social workers (postqualifying education and continuing professional development [CPD]). I used the skills and experience from two decades' group working with service users (the British term for *clients*) to inform my leadership of training groups.

Coleadership is common in the United Kingdom, for group work with service users and for training workshops with qualified social workers, and this has been my personal preference, too. My co-facilitator and I meet to plan the workshops, give immediate mutual feedback during the workshops, and debrief with each other following them. Often there is a period of travel after a day's workshops, or possibly an overnight stay if they take place over several days, and this is valuable time for reflection and feedback, following on soon after the actual experiences. This is an important lesson—the closer to the event you can debrief with a co-groupworker, the better; otherwise the rich detail quickly starts to fade.

Fruit salad

Group workers know that the chemistry of every group is unique; similarly, every workshop is different, depending on the participants. The membership differs from workshop to workshop, in terms of the personal biographies and values of the members and the particular mix of each group. Even so, there are some techniques that seem to benefit all groups, and one such activity is a warm-up toward the beginning of a group workshop. My coworker and I have become familiar with the use of a physical warm-up called Fruit Salad (I think it's sometimes referred to as *Fruit Basket* in North America). The group sits in a wide circle, and each person is assigned a fruit (the number of fruits depends on the number of participants, but you want at least four people in the same fruit group)—for example, apples, bananas, pears. The facilitator starts off in the middle of the group, without a seat, and calls out the name of one of the fruits, for example, pears, and all the pears must exchange seats, with the person in the middle also in the mix so that there is always one person remaining in the middle when all the chairs are filled. This person then goes on to shout a fruit—it can be a different fruit or the same as just called. The rules also allow the caller to shout "Fruit Salad!" in which case everybody must rise and find an alternative seat. In addition to the obvious benefits of fun and physical activity ahead of a day of largely cerebral and generally seated work, this warm-up is an interesting experiment in group learning. When "Fruit Salad" is called some people who are sat next to one another learn to swap seats—it's quite effective. And how long before the group as a whole learns (or somehow decides) to move just one seat along rather than scurrying across the middle of the circle? And will the group manage to decide which way it will move as a whole—clockwise or counterclockwise? There is much laughter as different sections of the group make different decisions at different times and move in different directions.

A change of plans

On this particular morning we are expecting 14 social workers for the workshop. We have their names in advance and see that there will be 11 women and three men, a fairly typical gender ratio. The participants begin to arrive for coffee, tea, and biscuits before the formal start. One of them arrives in a wheelchair.

My coworker and I are suddenly aware that we have never considered the possibility that there might be someone who is not physically able to leap out of a seat and run across the circle to claim another one. This, in itself, is important learning for us, but there is no time to reflect on that; for now, we must decide what we are going to do in fewer than 20 minutes' time, when we will begin the workshop. At the same time we must welcome and host newcomers and offer refreshments.

We manage to find some space to discuss what to do. We quickly agree that the obvious first option of having the wheelchair user included in the circle is not a safe one, in terms of people crashing into the chair as they rush across the circle; and, also, there would be no space for the wheelchair user to place her chair in another part of the circle because it's the people who move and not the chairs. The second option is not to use Fruit Salad. It would be a loss, but it's not essential to the day and no one would know it had gone. We've almost agreed on this when we sense that neither of us is happy with this solution, too quickly arrived at. The warm-up is really effective in pulling a group together, and it feels like a cop-out to abandon it. The pressure of time, it's now fewer than 15 minutes before everything starts, is pushing us toward an easy but instinctively unsatisfactory decision. My coworker goes to pour some more tea and welcome the still-arriving participants, and I ponder some more.

"What if Marian [the wheelchair user] has the role of 'caller'?" We discuss this as an option, looking at how it might work and how it might be perceived. It gives Marian a singular role in the group, but a powerful one. It does mark her difference (in this one dimension of physical ability) from the beginning but in a way that we hope is respectful, even powerful. Having decided this possible option, we agree that one of us should talk with Marian to see what she thinks about it and, as I am the person who usually introduces Fruit Salad, I go to speak with her.

Marian and I had spoken briefly when I first offered refreshments. Now I have to deal with what I realize is my own discomfort in confronting so early on (as I saw it) her difference from others in the group, and that includes me and my coworker. We are all able bodied, and she is disabled. The goal I have for myself is to frame the situation as a new one, rather than as a problem. I explain the Fruit Salad activity, both the rationale and the mechanics. I speak about the role of the caller a couple of times and Marian takes the cue and it is she who says, "Well, perhaps I could be the caller? I'd like that."

The activity goes really well. Marian and wheelchair form part of the circle, she calls out the fruits (and an occasional "Fruit Salad" for extra mayhem) and the group rush and whizz around her. There is a lot of fun with everyone holding on to Marian's call—she teases the group occasionally by taking a few seconds to build the tension. At the end of the game (there is no fixed end, the group workers just have to decide when they feel the time is right) I ask the group to reflect on the value of Fruit Salad, and any limitations, and why you might choose to use it with a group or not. Everyone is very positive, and many say they will be using it themselves in their own group work. No one mentions physical ability as a possible limitation. Often participants reflect that where they have ended up is not where they started, that they are literally in a different place, and this can give a quite different perspective on the group; on this occasion I observe that this is true for everyone except Marian and that in providing leadership for the group she has sacrificed this physical relocation. "Marian, would you like to change positions, we can easily make space here," says one of the participants, followed by a "mock competition" with various group members entreating Marian to ignore that offer and come to their part of the circle. She does wheel her chair so that she is in a different part of the circle, joking to the folks she leaves that it is nothing personal and that she fancies looking out of the window from the other side of the room.

What does this story tell us?

The first thing that struck me at the time was how easy it is "not" to think about diversity. I feel embarrassed that I had never considered person who is disabled taking part in the training. This was a failure of imagination (and, therefore, empathy) on my part. I could imagine, and had imagined, a situation where there might be one person in the group whose ethnicity or gender was different from all the rest of the group (perhaps because this was not infrequently the case), but Marian helped me to remember the *diversity* of diversity; that diversity is not code for race, ethnicity, or any one particular difference, and that difference has many expressions.

The Fruit Salad story also tells me that it is very easy for diversity to be problematized. We tell ourselves to celebrate diversity, yet how often do we actually see it as a difficulty, an obstacle, something to be managed; and a common consequence is to ignore difference and make subtle changes that we pretend are accommodating the differences but are really attempts to avoid them (in the Fruit Salad case, avoidance would have been achieved by abandoning the game).

The next lesson is how easy it is to fall into the trap of making solutions *for* other people rather than *with* them. My coworker and I thought we had found a way forward that was inclusive, but it was our way forward and not necessarily Marian's. With the best of intentions, we can behave in ways that are patronizing because they exclude people from the *process* of arriving at an inclusive decision. As it happens, Marian's thinking leapfrogs ours and she makes the suggestion herself. Another of my reflections is how very subtle and delicate these issues are, perhaps particularly so in the British cultural context where communications are often indirect and *sotto voce*. It's not about "dumping" the decision on another person ("Marian, what shall we do?"), and it's also not about making decisions for others ("Marian, don't worry, here's what we do"). It's about sharing and negotiating responsibility together. Including people in the process is a sound overall principle, but might Marian be pleased that the group facilitators have done some preparatory work and thinking and can offer the beginnings of a suggestion? Is this, then, an appropriate use of the group leaders' power and responsibility?

An important principle of good groupwork practice is involving the group in decision making. It is a good principle. But the Fruit Salad story highlights the significance of timing when applying this principle. To have invited the group at the beginning of the workshop to consider how to include Marian in Fruit Salad would have been crass and put a sharp, unkind spotlight on her. This is often why diversity is not discussed, because highlighting the diversity seems to problematize it. However, just because silence may be appropriate at one moment does not mean that it continues to be appropriate. When the workshop group was comfortable with itself, at the performing stage one might say, it was possible to return the group's reflection on the activity; by now, Marian was no longer defined by her disability, "a wheelchair user: (or even worse, "*The*" wheelchair user, somehow emblematic of all her "kind," which is the basis of stereotyping). She was better known to the group as *Marian*, a much more complex sum of all the relationships she had made in the group, just as this was true of all the other members of the group—no longer "'able-bodied people," but Suranne, Tom, Tanya, and so on. This included us, no longer just "the group leaders" but Mark and Catherine. The group could take its own learning from the experience and reflect on it.

Visible and invisible differences

The story makes me think about the difference between visible and invisible differences. Marian's physical disability was clearly visible because she used a wheelchair, but what if she had an arthritic condition that was not evident? Or, if she had been visibly very obese, would we have—should we have—made an assumption about her level of ability to take part in a fast-moving physical activity? We can think of other differences, such as sexuality, that are not necessarily visible and that might or might not be disclosed during the course of a group.

I hesitated to tell this story, as it did not seem to convey sufficient ambition when considering the breadth and depth of the topic of diversity, especially the political and power dimension of oppressed minorities. However, my hesitation was overcome by what happened right at the end of the group when participants were leaving. Marian approached my coworker and me to thank us for Fruit Salad, saying that she really enjoyed it. She seemed quite emotional as she told us that she'd found the experience "moving" (an especially poignant word in the circumstances) and that most of the time her experience has been that her disability is ignored and not taken any account of. So, the final lesson for me was that "small" acts are often not that small.

Ultimately, learning comes from stepping outside our comfort zones and taking risks. Using an activity like Fruit Salad involves some small degree of risk: a risk that some people won't enjoy it; a risk that they won't "get it"; a risk that someone might stumble and have an injury; a risk that there will be one member of the group who, for some seen or unseen reason, cannot take part. Group leaders have a responsibility to guide their group through risk taking, to embrace diversity rather than abandon it, and to develop the confidence that they—and the group—will not always get it right.

Hope and Sorrow

Joshua L. Miller

I was training a group of about 20 farmers, religious leaders, teachers, and local officials in psychosocial capacity building in the wake of a 22-year armed conflict involving the Lords Resistance Army (LRA). We were in a small, hot, humid room in a small, isolated village in the bush, which happened to be the village where Joseph Kony, the leader of the LRA, was from. It was the last day of 4 days of training with an incredibly engaged and attentive group of people. The hope was that they would then share what they had learned with other people who were not at the workshop. When they listed the problems that they are encountering in their community they stressed land disputes, domestic violence, alcoholism, and suicide. I discussed with them how these are often symptoms of trauma after an armed conflict and proceeded to talk about the neurobiology of trauma, psychological, and emotional symptoms and behavioral consequences. After describing things like flashbacks and intrusive images I asked if in their work with others in the community they could offer any examples of encountering people with trauma.

Of course all of the participants in the workshop, like everyone living in Northern Uganda, personally experienced the horrors of surviving the armed conflict. A significant number of men in the group had large, deep, and sometimes disfiguring scars on their necks, faces, and heads. Two people talked about how they were afraid of and triggered by certain places where LRA attacks and massacres had taken place. Many people in the group nodded as they spoke.

A woman in her fifties or sixties wearing a purple dress and a white headscarf then stood and spoke. The room became silent and somber as the woman sat down and buried her face in her hands. When I asked my translator, a man in his twenties, what she had said, he could not speak and began to cry. I asked him if he wanted to sit down and he nodded and turned toward the back of the room. I asked one of my cotrainers and a friend, an Acholi Catholic Priest named Father Remigio to stand next to me and describe what the woman had said. He proceeded to tell me a story with atrocities involving children so horrific that I will not share it here.

I have heard many heartbreaking narratives in my work, but it was all I could do to remain composed, and turned to the woman and thanked her for her courage in sharing her story, acknowledging how painful it must have been to not only witness this but also to recount it to us. I then turned to the group and said that the stories that had been shared illustrated how everyone in the area had been exposed to such distressing violence that the question was not whether people had experienced trauma but rather how profound their trauma was and how long it had lasted.

I asked Father Remigio, who was still standing next to me, if he would speak to the group about what can help people to recover from trauma, anticipating what he would say from our many conversations and work together about this topic. In Acholi he talked about the importance of people sharing their stories—whether by speech, writing, drama, song, or dance—drawing on cultural traditions and community support, and how after even the most dreadful experiences and catastrophic losses, people could eventually heal and even encounter joy. I asked him if he could ask someone in the group to lead us in an Acholi mourning song. The woman who shared the story stood, followed by everyone else in the room. She then started clapping her hands rhythmically and stamping her feet and singing, which everyone else in the room joined, with a call and response. While we were all swaying and clapping, she began to dance, other women whooped in high-pitched shrieks. The woman began to smile, waving her hands in the air as people clapped for her. Finally she waved us to a halt, and everyone went outside where lunch had just been delivered.

When we returned and I asked the group what they thought helped people to heal from trauma she was the first to speak and said in Acholi, "I think that crying helps." I asked her if she thought that the tears cleanse a deep hidden wound, and she nodded. An hour later a monsoon struck, turning the muddy red roads into rivers and forcing us all to huddle in the middle of the room where it was still dry. Some chickens sheltered in the doorway. The rain cleared, and at the close of the workshop the woman again stood and led us in another dance/song, one that reflected the strength, hope, and aspirations of the Acholi people.

To a Classroom in Botswana (and Back) in Search of Cultural Understanding

Amy Nitza

Culture hides much more than it reveals and strangely enough what it hides, it hides most effectively from its own participants. Years of study have convinced me that the real job is not to understand foreign cultures, but to understand our own. (Hall, 1959, pp. 29–30)

I was first exposed to this quote only after having spent a year teaching and conducting research at the University of Botswana as a Fulbright Scholar. I found the quote when doing background reading in preparation for teaching a multicultural counseling course for the first time. I was struck enough by it to place it at the top of the syllabus for the course, the first and only time I have ever used a quote to frame an entire course. The quote was powerful for me because it put words to many of my experiences living, teaching, and working in another culture for a year that I had not yet been able to pull together with coherence. It provided a frame for the experiences I wanted students in my course to be able to have.

My journey to this point started several years earlier when I accompanied one of my former professors to assist in facilitating a week-long group counseling workshop in Botswana. It was my first time teaching in an international context, and I was equal parts excited and curious. The structure and content of the workshop were standard group counseling training fare. By most accounts, it was a success. Over the course of the week, students became engaged with each other, with the facilitators, and with the content. They listened carefully, and many of them took the risk of trying out their skills as group leaders during role plays. The end of the week brought a lively closure celebration with singing, dancing, and exchanging of contact information.

Yet there was a disconnect. I could feel it, but I could not name it. Throughout the workshop, it seemed to me that there were times when the participants were hearing something different than what the facilitators were trying to communicate. The facilitators knew their stuff, no question about it. And the participants were professionals who had been hand-picked to attend the training, several of them having traveled for 2 days, some of that by foot, to get there. These were bright and committed people who were eager to learn. Nevertheless, I was aware that the impact of the workshop was not exactly what was intended. Something was getting "lost in translation."

Clearly the disconnect was cultural. But what specifically was this cultural disconnect? And how could it be addressed? My curiosity was heightened, and I decided as I processed these questions that the only way for me to find answers was to immerse myself more fully in the culture and understand it more deeply. In doing so, perhaps I could find ways to bridge the gaps that I had noticed in the workshop.

Two years later, I was back in the country as a Fulbright Scholar, eager to explore the answers to the questions that had arisen for me in the original workshop. Those questions had shaped my Fulbright proposal and the goals for my project. In the United States, we know a great deal about groups. We know not only that they work, but a great deal about "how" they work. In other words, we have a solid understanding of the group processes and change mechanisms that help make groups effective, as well as of the interventions that group leaders can use to facilitate these processes and mechanisms. However, these outcomes, processes, and interventions are all set primarily in a Western cultural paradigm; little had been written at that point (at least in Western literature) about how all of these things apply, or don't, in other countries and cultures across the world. With the hypothesis that group interventions, when applied effectively to the cultural context of Botswana, have the potential power to be effective in addressing a number of psychosocial issues facing people in that country, I set out to explore how Western group theory and practice could best be adapted to do so. The journey that began as I arrived in the country and began to make a plan for operationalizing my ideas was bumpier, deeper, and more meaningful than I anticipated. In some ways, the journey also left me with more questions than answers, which perhaps is the best outcome of at all. In any case, I learned much along the way.

Processes of personal growth and cultural awareness

As expected, I was assigned to teach a group counseling course to graduate students, something I had done many times at home. However, despite my command of the subject from a Western perspective, I found myself being very hesitant in delivering the content. What began as an awareness that all the concepts I was introducing would likely not translate directly into this context developed into an experience of questioning everything I "knew," even as I was teaching it.

This experience of beginning to question everything, and the resulting sense of disequilibrium that occurred, was heightened by some important contextual factors. By 2008 Botswana, along with much of the rest of Southern Africa, had been suffering from the worst of the world-wide

HIV/AIDS epidemic for nearly a decade (Joint United Nations Programme on HIV/AIDS & World Health Organization, 2008). Despite a massive international response that included money and expertise, it was becoming clear to people in the middle of the crisis there that this response had to some extent missed the mark. Conversations with my Batswana colleagues (*Batswana* is the term used to refer to the people of Botswana) indicated that they perceived this to be due to a lack of, or inadequate, cultural understanding. They experienced this cultural insensitivity on the part of outsiders as reminiscent of the colonization that their country had overcome within the past 50 years. Thus, their reactions to international "experts" coming in with new ideas were understandably strong and skeptical. For example, one colleague, when asked by an American researcher to help her norm an American depression screening instrument for use in in Botswana, stated "We don't want your Western instrument; help us develop our own." With this backdrop to my work, I became even more cautious about being culturally appropriate in all that I did, to the extent that I often felt paralyzed and as if I shouldn't act at all.

As the group counseling course continued, I worked my way through these hesitations and slowly began to reestablish a new, different, and more culturally informed equilibrium. This happened in several ways. First, the classroom itself developed into a cohesive working group, and as it did I observed the group process occurring much as it does in many other settings. Although the students were familiar with each other before the semester started, most of their other courses were not structured in ways that welcomed or even allowed them to share their own ideas and experiences in the classroom. Their initial hesitation to doing so was strong; they appeared to me to be much more reluctant to engage with each other than my students at home, due to cultural traditions in and outside of the classroom. Through experiential exercises that encouraged them to begin to take risks in self-disclosing around "safe" topics, they began to overcome their initial hesitation. As they began to identify with each other's experiences, this cascaded into further attempts to take risks in sharing and connecting. Observing this transformation in a group that had such cultural inhibitions in doing so allowed me to begin to "trust the process" of group development. As I did so, I was able to more comfortably, and meaningfully, explore other cultural factors as they arose. In academic terms, perhaps seeing the group process develop allowed me to identify some universal aspects of groups that were not culturally dependent. Once I was able to work with these familiar concepts, I felt more grounded, and it was easier for me to be able to explore the culturally relative aspects of groups as they occurred.

A second means by which I was able to develop a new cultural equilibrium occurred as I got to know the students as individuals, which allowed me to move beyond the initial experience of being an outsider in a culturally homogeneous group of students. For example, as we talked about the power of universality, one student described the shame and isolation he experienced due to his stutter. This led to another student sharing her pain as a mother in watching how her child was socially rejected for being albino (a condition traditionally linked to witchcraft in Botswana). In a discussion about goal setting in groups, a student who was also a Catholic priest shared his dream of opening a school for the orphans in his home village, and another discussed the personal mission she had to improve conditions for the blind children at the school in which she taught. As we all connected as a group of unique individuals through this sharing, trust and cohesion within the classroom group deepened, and we were all increasingly able to take risks and share observations and reactions. This level of safety was key to deepening my cultural awareness and exploration. Just as the students became increasingly able to take risks in sharing personal dreams and concerns, I felt increasingly safe enough to make observations and ask questions when I noticed potential cultural differences, and to use these as a basis for richer discussion.

A final factor was my awareness that because the students were a culturally homogenous group functioning within their own culture, they themselves were not necessarily aware of the cultural influences on their own thinking and interpersonal behavior. As Hall (1959) described, their own culture hid as much from them as mine had from me. This awareness allowed me to overcome some of my hesitations about teaching concepts that might be inconsistent with their culture. Instead, as a group we developed a process by which I would introduce course concepts, and then together we would explore their reactions to those concepts, including but not limited to the ways the concepts fit or did not with their cultural experiences.

One particularly powerful discussion involved the influence of cultural beliefs and practices around gender. As we discussed the impact of advice giving in groups and cultural differences in the use of advice, the conversation shifted to the authoritarian role of the paternal uncle in many Batswana families. Students explained that traditionally, uncles have the authority to make important decisions for family members, and particularly women, that cannot necessarily be challenged. As I shared my unfamiliarity with this family structure and contrasted it that which might be found in the United States, students began to explore this for themselves. Their exploration led to a larger discussion about the often rigid gender roles within their culture. It appeared that for some students, this was the first time they had considered the limiting effect of gender on their behavior; it seemed to help them name and consider previously unexplored cultural influences on their lives and ultimately resulted in a rich discussion of how these influences might affect the group process. In this way, we learned together about our own cultures at the same time that we were learning about the culture of each other.

Cultural influences on group dynamics

The personal and cultural growth experiences that I had as an instructor occurred in tandem with the academic exploration I undertook to answer my original questions about the translation of Western group counseling to the cultural context of Botswana. The rich discussion that developed within the classroom generated important research questions in this regard. Perhaps the biggest set of questions that arose involved the role of group counseling within a collective culture. My original hypothesis had been that group interventions make much more sense than individual interventions in such a culture. It seemed reasonable that group-based interventions could be particularly beneficial in collectivist settings in which individuals' identities are tied so closely to that of their "group." However, my observations and conversations with students made it clear that the issue is more complex. For example, self-exploration and reflection, which are hallmarks of the group counseling process, did not necessarily seem to be emphasized in the collectivist culture of the Batswana, in which priority is traditionally given to interpersonal obligations over individual needs. In a counseling group that is a microcosm of a collectivist worldview are individual group members able to feel comfortable and free to explore their individual needs and experiences?

A related set of questions involves the group interventions that might be most valuable in facilitating members' personal growth in such groups. Communication among collectivist peoples such as the Batswana tend to be high context communication patterns in which much of what is communicated is done indirectly through the context surrounding a conversation. Direct verbal communication involving disagreement, confrontation, and/or assertiveness are limited. How then do group interventions that draw heavily from the individualist and low-context communication style of the West operate in such groups? For example, interpersonal feedback exchange involves sharing of personal observations and reactions to each other. Can such an intervention be effective in groups made up of members with high-context communication styles?

A final set of questions arose around the process of group development. The creation of a cohesive, productive, and therapeutic group climate typically occurs as the group moves through a series of predictable stages. Based on what I had observed about communication within their culture, it seemed clear that the processes and stages that a homogeneous group of Batswana would go through to develop a productive and healing group climate would be to some degree unique to that culture. I was, and remain, convinced that there are aspects of the group process that are universally healing. However, I became less clear about what these universal processes might actually be. What are the characteristics of a productive and healing group climate within this specific culture? Which elements of it are culturally bound? What are the stages that a group might go through to develop such a climate and how similar or different are those stages to those described in Western literature?

Each of these sets of questions that arose for me through experience and observation are important considerations as the field of group counseling continues to advance its application in multicultural and international settings. There is an urgent need for more empirical investigation on these and other questions in order to guide the work of teachers and practitioners around the world.

Conclusion

"We are most likely to become aware of our cultural assumptions when they are violated or when we are plunged into cultural settings different from those that we are used to" (Gielen, Draguns, & Fish, 2008, p. 5). My experiences teaching group counseling in a setting very different from my own allowed me to have my cultural assumptions violated in beneficial ways. Professionally, I was successful in at least beginning my quest to learn more about the culture of Botswana and generating potential answers to my questions about how to adapt Western group counseling to this context.

At the same time, I went through a personal process of losing my footing and feeling frozen out of concern for being culturally sensitive, and then working my way back to a new equilibrium through my relationships and interactions with students. This process, which was more difficult than I had anticipated, has had an ongoing impact on my teaching back in the United States. Within the classroom, I now seek to provide activities and other opportunities for previously hidden aspects of students' own culture and its impact on them to be revealed and experienced. My journey to Botswana and back has convinced me that allowing students to experience some sense of disequilibrium and then facilitating multiple reflection and processing opportunities for them to put the pieces back together again in a new way is essential to developing cultural understanding among people and groups.

References

Gielen, U. P., Draguns, J. G., & Fish, J. M. (2008). Principles of multicultural counseling and therapy: An introduction. In U. P. Gielen, J. G. Draguns, & J. M. Fish (Eds.), *Principles of multicultural counseling and therapy* (pp. 1–34). New York, NY: Routledge.

Hall, E. T. (1959). *The silent language.* New York, NY: Doubleday.

Joint United Nations Programme on HIV/AIDS & World Health Organization. (2008). *Epidemiological fact sheet on HIV and AIDS: Botswana 2008 update.* Retrieved from http://apps.who.int/globalatlas/predefinedReports/EFS2008/full/EFS2008_BW.pdf

Exploring Personal and Professional Understanding of Nonmonogamous Relationships: Reflections on a Group Work–Informed Workshop

Sarah R. Hemphill, Shirley R. Simon, and Brandon Haydon

In contemporary Western society, monogamous marriage is considered the ideal, with any relationships deviating from this standard viewed as non-normative and taboo. Yet the prevalence of nonmonogamous relationships is increasingly irrefutable. *Nonmonogamy* is defined as relationships or actions that deviate from the norm of a traditional two-person exclusive partnership, often designating concurrent involvement or pursuit of multiple romantic or sexual relationships. Given today's political climate of espoused "family values," marital legal rights, and the sanctity of the normative marriage structure, addressing nonmonogamy is risky, fraught with value-laden judgments and personal assumptions. To address this topic in a public form is in itself a risky endeavor; however that is exactly what we, three graduate students and a faculty advisor, undertook.

Although sexual identity and marital status are both protected by the National Association of Social Workers Code of Ethics (2008), we knew that many practitioners have yet to examine their understanding or question their biases around relationship identities. The simple mention of the non-monogamous relationships to social work colleagues frequently elicited awkward pauses and a sense of discomfort, as well as narratives of personal pain from nonconsensual infidelity (cheating) and fear of domestic abuse or power imbalances under polygamy. It was the need to confront this discomfort and lack of awareness that propelled us forward to create a group-centered workshop on this topic. Our commitment to serve vulnerable populations proved more powerful than our fears. The International Association of Social Work with Groups (IASWG) Symposium provided a space to begin this conversation.

Asking social work professionals to explore their understandings and biases about topics like nonmonogamy can be challenging. We knew we needed to create a safe, nonjudgmental space, with a nondidactic, participatory environment. We began the workshop with a brief definition of *nonmonogamy*; invited participants to share their motivations for attending; facilitated an icebreaker exploring the concept of attraction; distributed a handout with terms, visuals, and resources; divided into small discussion groups; and closed with a large open-ended group discussion.

During the first few minutes of the workshop we could feel the awkwardness and tension—nervous laughter and hushed whispers. This was especially evident as we shared examples of nonmonogamy, including "open relationships" in which a couple sanctions sexual and/or romantic relationships outside of the partnership; polyamory, where individuals or couples are able to love multiple people at the same time; and other arrangements such as "triads" in which groups of three (or more) people are in a relationship with one another. The group members opened up about their reasons for coming to the workshop, and some participants "confessed" a lack of knowledge, volunteering that they had never heard of terms like "polyamory." Others, however, self-identified as living in polyamorous marriages and families. As the workshop progressed, we felt the group relax, becoming more willing to share and question.

Guided by handouts identifying and defining relevant terms such as "family" and "jealousy" as well as more topic-specific terms such as "compersion"[1] and "metamour,"[2] participants felt safe enough to ask the group to clarify definitions, discussing concepts like what "cheating," "commitment," and "attraction" really meant to each of us.

For one small group, conversation was centered on the notion of "commitment." Members explored past experiences of what it meant to be in a committed relationship. They examined assumptions garnered from predominant societal traditions and family narratives that they had seldom explicitly labeled or discussed. Members raised questions about flirting or fantasizing, beginning to see that assumed norms were seldom universal. For instance, they grappled with questions such as "Is it acceptable to flirt with others if you have no intention of pursuing a further connection?" "Are fantasies about exes allowed?" Participants were able to acknowledge and hear one another describe their assumptions about commitment; for one person it started with the first kiss, whereas for another it was after a certain amount of time and emotional investment. Some were even able to disclose instances when they felt uncertain whether they had violated the shared commitment within their relationships. One group member shared her ambivalence about having remained in contact with her old boyfriend, whereas another questioned at what point it was no longer appropriate to continue checking his online dating profile after meeting someone new. Each small group discussion focused on different issues, but all explored relationship diversity on a personal as well as intellectual level.

By the closing large-group discussion, we could all feel an almost tangible sense of community and comfort, having safely explored a controversial topic, with many participants addressing concepts not usually verbalized. Participants felt reluctant to end the discussion, and many stayed talking beyond the formal conclusion of the workshop.

Facilitator reflections

I first realized the need for professionals to be better informed about non-monogamy while I was working in reproductive health. I remember the shame women carried whenever there was a question about sexual partners —not because they regretted their actions, but because they expected to be judged or look down upon for having chosen a less societally sanctioned way to experience their sexuality. I noticed a hesitancy when clients disclosed relationships that included bringing close friends into the bedroom, multiple anonymous partners, loving and committed groups of adults, or sex workers who did not let their careers get in the way of a committed partnership, as well as many other variants of romantic and sexual connections. Although socially diverse, all of these clients carried the common expectation that professionals could shame and discriminate against their decisions to physi-cally, romantically, or emotionally connect with more than one person. As I have grown as a social worker, my clients have continued to show me that there are many ways people can express love. And, just as we would not expect there to be one racial, gendered, or sexual identity, to expect the norm of the traditional married couple to fit everyone denies so much of our clients' lived experiences.

In working with and acknowledging nonmonogamous clients, we see that they are seeking therapy and joining groups for a wide variety of reasons that may not be related to their relationships or relationship choices. This is why it pains me to hear professionals inadvertently dismiss or shame this popula-tion, because as many individuals who are nonmonogamous are closeted in their social and professional lives, it is likely that these same social workers unknowingly encounter clients who are nonmonogamous regularly in their professional practice.

Group workers have long been advocates for diversity and self-determination. So, as I prepared the workshop on nonmonogamy, I was grateful that it would be a room full of group workers to whom we would be presenting this personal and controversial topic. Yet I was still nervous to push the boundaries of cultural competence beyond the standard acknowl-edgement of sexual orientation, focusing on a population that is frequently condemned as "perverted," "promiscuous," and antithetical to "natural family structure." I was especially afraid to offend or disappoint the faculty members I looked up to as mentors. What assumptions would they make about my marriage? Would the people I respect write me off as "too radical"? Are there some populations that my profession is just not ready to serve?

Fortunately, these prepresentation jitters did not deter me or my copre-senters. As group workers, I feel we share a responsibility to continue a tradition of advocacy for social justice. Once the group began to engage with the topic, I soon saw that the participants were eager to learn about this population, and the majority of judgments or negative assumptions came from a lack of knowledge that gave way to curiosity rather than moral rigidity. Individuals could have easily dismissed our message as "taboo," irrelevant to their work, or not worthy of the time and emotional investment needed to foster understanding, but entering this exploration with other likeminded peers promoted a sense of safety and understanding that facilitated engagement. My cofacilitators and I came to appreciate how the same principles of mutual aid, universalization, and social justice that allow group workers to support vulnerable populations can also be used to create a foundation to explore culturally sensitive topics. Just as I hope to support and empower my nonmonogamous clients, I found it similarly important to support and empower the professionals engaging in such a value-laden exploration. As participants began to grapple with more difficult questions, owning their own vulnerabilities, biases and lack of knowledge, it was evident that our focus on empowerment and mutual aid supported members in becoming more open.

I was thrilled with how well participants responded to the workshop. I felt that they were leaving with a foundation to further explore their understanding of nonmonogamy, having taken the first steps in building this cultural competence. If anything, I had underestimated the need for this workshop and the kindness and open mindedness that my fellow group workers would bring to exploring this controversial topic. Confidence and compassion can be contagious. Although participants left expressing how empowered they felt to begin to speak with clients about alternative relationships, I left feeling empowered to continue speaking with other professionals about this population that is underacknowledged and marginalized. Given this experience, I feel even more committed to increasing opportunities to foster discussions on nonmonogamy with the larger professional community.

Faculty advisor reflections

When several of my students proposed submitting an abstract to present a workshop based on group work principles to explore social workers' understanding of clients in nonmonogamous, polyamorous, or romantically and/or sexually open relationships, I had a multitude of responses. I was enthusiastic because I knew that this is an underexplored topic that merits attention, and because I knew that IASWG is a supportive, encouraging professional community that would be open to such a presentation. I also trusted in the maturity and professional abilities of these particular MSW students to carry it off well. I knew that the students had taken a group work course and were cognizant of the importance of group work principles.

On the other hand, as a relatively traditional professional who has been in a monogamous relationship for more than 40 years, I also experienced some trepidation about my comfort level and role in encouraging and participating in this workshop. How did I feel about my name being affiliated with this topic? What would my colleagues and administrators at a religiously based academic institution think about this? As I interacted with the students, listened to their plans for the workshop, and reflected on my own personal and professional values, I was reassured and excited about the potential impact of the presentation. I dialogued with the facilitators about the importance of utilizing group work principles to create a group experience that would encourage open discussion and exploration.

I experienced pride in observing the group work skill that the student facilitators employed in leading the session. They began the workshop with a clear statement of purpose and a confident, inviting demeanor. They established a group contract incorporating issues of confidentiality, mutual respect, and nonjudgmental interaction and encouraged trust with their calm, nonauthoritarian personas. The leaders successfully created a safe participatory environment that facilitated engagement and interaction while also managing time and being cognizant of the likely limitations on the depth of vulnerability prevalent in this one-time group. They responded to questions and challenges nondefensively, relinquishing power and control to the group members whenever possible. For instance, when a participant asked whether "polyamory (romantic consensual non-monogamy) is socially irresponsible in the age of STIs (sexually transmitted infections) and HIV," the facilitators shared their knowledge of the literature as well as their professional experiences but also encouraged responses and feedback from the participants. They created an esprit of mutual aid within the small groups, asking for participants' personal and professional perspectives on issues of nonmonogamy.

As the session unfolded, I observed other "traditional" long-term colleagues ask questions about terminology, safety precautions, feelings of jealousy, possessiveness, clinical responsibilities, and social taboos. Participants, including myself, began to look at long-held values from a more open position. Although this was certainly only a beginning, attendees did seem to leave the session more informed and willing to look at issues of nonmonogamy through a more open, nonjudgmental lens. On a personal level, I took away a greater willingness to explore nontraditional attitudes and practices that differed from my own choices. I gained language and understanding to be able to better discuss nonmonogamy. I left the session with many new thoughts and perspectives that will inform my personal and professional interactions.

Follow-up note: My experience of being able to explore this topic within a safe, well-led group convinced me that this workshop should be replicated at our home institution. Feedback from the written evaluations and follow-up conversations with participants supported this decision. I was able to arrange for the facilitators to lead a similar session as an extracurricular offering the following fall. The presentation was very well attended despite the lack of academic incentives and seemed to address a topic of interest to many. Again, the participants' responses were consistently positive with many requests for follow-up sessions and discussions. The attendance and the effectiveness of both workshop offerings affirmed the need for more group interactions on this important topic. Being affiliated with this presentation was a meaningful personal and professional undertaking that increased my awareness of the need for further dialogue and discussion.

Conclusion

For us, this has been a meaningful journey of personal and professional exploration and growth. Our experience reinforces the need for social workers and other professionals to explore their own personal and professional understanding of non-monogamy. We hope for and encourage the replication of this workshop across multiple settings.

Acknowledgment

The authors wish to recognize Natalie A. Hock for her role as a facilitator and contributor to the development of the workshop.

Notes

1. A feeling of pleasure from witnessing one's partner's pleasure, often viewed as the opposite of jealousy.
2. One's partner's partner, for example, my husband's boyfriend is my metamour.

GROWING UP

"I did not know then that this is what life is - just when you master the geometry of one world, it slips away, and suddenly again, you're swarmed by strange shapes and impossible angles."

Ta-Nehisi Coates

Which Drums Should We Play?

Katrina Skewes McFerran ⓘD

As a music therapist, I have faith in the power of music to transcend the differences between people and provide a way for people to come together in unison. There is an enormous amount of theory and research that sits behind my beliefs, and an understanding that this can only occur when the circumstances are right; but I do believe it. So it was challenging for me to be confronted by the realization that music can also reinforce the divides between people. My experiences also provided an important reminder that each of the various strategies in my well-travelled toolkit fails some of the time.

The school where these realizations occurred comprises a diverse cohort of students, with more than 60 nationalities represented in the student body of 400 young people. These figures confirmed what was already apparent when I walked around the school. A wide range of skin colors was evident in the schoolyard, and the culturally diverse ways of relating were almost equally apparent. The school buildings were dull and grey, but there was more than enough life and energy coming from the young people to counter the flatness of the landscape.

My role in the school was to create a flourishing music culture that would promote connectedness and well-being. I was to spend one day each week in the school working with teachers, students, families, community musicians, and anyone else who was willing to be involved in music. It was an experiment in sustainability to see whether I could share my music therapy knowledge in a meaningful way with the school and then leave. I was confident that something could be achieved and equally prepared to not know exactly what that might be, so walking around and observing was an important part of getting to know the school.

The contrast between the sterile grey buildings and the energy of older boys in the school was one of the first things that caught my attention. These young men were around age 14 and 15 years, and most of them stood at least a few inches taller than me in stature. Some had a slightly wild look in their eyes, and some looked a little downtrodden. But most of them were constantly on the move, roaming about as though they didn't quite know where they were going during the lunch break, or bouncing up and down in their seats during class. Some were from Arabic backgrounds, some were from the Pacific, others were from Asia, and the occasional Eastern European and other Anglo-Saxon varieties were also present.

After speaking with the school principal and the well-being coordinator I began to think that engaging these young men in school could be an important focus for achieving connectedness. Few of them were flourishing in the strict school culture that had been enforced as a way of ensuring violence did not result from the clash of cultures in the school. A zero-tolerance approach to behavior meant that many of these active young men were frequently in trouble and there were few opportunities for them to shine. My previous experiences as a music therapist suggested that working with drums might provide us with the opportunities we needed.

"Drums have a marvelous capacity to get very loud."

I was humbled to discover that the well-being coordinator had already had the same idea and had been experimenting with a structured drumming program that was meant to improve self-confidence and positive interactions. A small group of teachers were keen to explore the activity further and to build on the drumming skills they had already gained through professional development workshops. I could see that it would take some work to move beyond the highly organized approach they were trialing and toward a more creative use of the drums for expression and encounter. However, I thought it would be critical to do so, because I perceived too many negative repercussions if the young men were not able or willing to play together in time. The same pattern of playful behavior that was already resulting in restrictive responses was likely to occur. Drums have a marvelous capacity to get very loud, and adults have an equally spectacular ability to get scared or annoyed by the sounds they create.

The first time we tried to play together was exactly as I had predicted. Despite my best attempts to prepare the teachers for a flexible approach to playing, the experience quickly spiraled beyond their comfort zone. I thought it would be safe enough to begin with a call-and-response exercise, and I played a short riff that the group tried to copy me back. Hit the drum twice, pause, they copy; hit the drum three times, pause, they copy. It was chaos, as it always is in the beginning of such games. But when a music therapist is facilitating the group it isn't about getting it right, it's about listening to one another and being engaged together. It can be these moments of chaos during which differences are transcended and everybody leans in, trying to get it right and laughing as they get it wrong. But that wasn't exactly how it went on this day.

The teachers stayed with me when I was in the lead, but they began to struggle when I passed the leadership on to the other group members. The first boy tried to play something, and the group found it difficult to hear the rhythm in what he was doing. There was laughter as I encouraged everyone to persist. The second boy had a natural sense of rhythm but played a riff that was too long and too complex. More laughing. Once again, I knew this was perfectly normal and encouraged us all to keep focused without trying to reduce the energy levels. We moved around the circle and everyone revealed something of themselves through their attempts to play. Some could not overcome their fear of failure, and so we moved past them. Others could not stop once they had started. Some were loud. Some were inaudible.

By the end of the exercise, the cofacilitating teachers had had enough. One of the well-being leaders decided to step in and establish some sense of control. She asked the group to learn a rhythm from her so that everyone could play together in time. I agreed that there are many benefits to playing in synchrony but wondered whether the group would actually be able to achieve it. A fantastic drum circle leader can get any group to play together in a matter of moments, but the novice, especially one who is lacking in confidence, less easily achieves it. What an expert musician will do is to play with such gusto and accuracy that it is hard to miss the beat. Like a charismatic speaker, the great drummer can draw the crowd in so that they barely notice what their hands are doing.

"I could see that being too flexible was too much for the adults."

The teacher did not have the skills to draw the group in, and as she stopped to correct herself and then told the group to wait while she tried again, it was my turn to feel tension levels rising. I could see that being too flexible was too much for the adults, and I knew from experience that being too strict with drums requires either musical charisma or a well-established hierarchy. My mind raced wildly as I tried to think of compromises that we could make. I could take a stronger leadership role and support the teacher, but my leadership style is always quite loose and I knew from experience that being strict doesn't always work for me. I knew I couldn't reassert my leadership and start my old activity again, because that would over-ride the hierarchy of the school and it would seem I was siding with the group members against the adults. Another error. As I watched and contemplated, I grasped on to the idea of getting the young men to share drum patterns from their cultural heritage. Many of the young men had been playing particular rhythms when they had their turn at leading the group, so I knew they could play. I had talked with the teachers about drumming being a way to work with diverse cultures, so it wouldn't be completely new. I decided to give it a shot.

As the "playing together" exercise ground to a halt, I called out my suggestion. I pointed to one of the Arabic boys and asked if he could play us a rhythm that he knew from his family. He looked gleeful, then a little nervous, and then, like the teacher, he stumbled and had to make a number of attempts to play it out. Another one of the boys called out that he could do it better, and I turned the attention of the group toward him. This one had no sense of rhythm however and just hit the drum fast and loud, wanting the attention of the group. I then pointed to one of the young men of Maori origin and asked for a rhythm from his culture. Adopting a relaxed style, he slapped his hands on the drum and played something slow and groovy. Suddenly, the cultural war was on, and the different cultures were playing over the top of one another, shouting and claiming the superiority of their own style. The differences were striking, and even if they hadn't been calling out, the clash would have been apparent. The teachers looked at me in distress. I reluctantly raised my voice, and after a little while got the attention of the group again. Without looking at my fellow professionals, I played a very simple rhythm and encouraged everyone to join in. I conceded defeat in allowing the chaos to take over and used what musical charisma I had left to limp through to the end of the session.

"The lines of distinction between youth and adults had also been reinforced."

It took me a number of weeks and some good supervision to recognize what I had learned from this session. Even though drums are often a great way to bring young men together, in this case, they had reinforced the lines of power and control that existed at many levels in the school. Although there was a lot of enthusiasm to play the drums, they symbolized manhood and culture more than they represented possibilities for peace and connection across the dividing lines. The lines of distinction between adults and youth had also been reinforced, which was precisely the opposite of what I had hoped to achieve. As I let go of my own attachment to the drums as the perfect tool for working with active young men, I tried to imagine what else we could share.

I spent more time listening to the young people in the school, trying to identify if there were particular genres of music that might bridge the gaps. Some liked Rock, some liked Hip-Hop, some only liked the music of their own cultures, and some only liked music when it was playing in the background for their video games. Not drums, not style of music, not dancing, not singing. In the end, the answer came from an unexpected source. I was approached by a wise older woman as I stood waiting at the gate of my own children's school later that week. She wanted to tell me about a great new drummer she had met who ran a program called the Anti Racism Action Band in a nearby suburb. I took his number and promised to give him a call, though I had no idea what we were meant to talk about.

When we did speak, I found myself lamenting the situation I was in at the other school and describing the challenges of drumming. The drummer was interested to hear my reflections and also had a couple of suggestions he wanted me to consider. He had been experimenting with body percussion in his work with young people who came from poverty-filled backgrounds and couldn't access neither instruments nor the money for them. He claimed that body percussion was just as much fun as a drum circle but didn't require any resources, so they could do it anywhere once they got the hang of it. As I finished the phone call, I was filled with a sense of possibility for the school as well as some selfish pleasure for myself. It had been a while since I got a new idea for my toolkit and I could see that this might be a new avenue for growth and discovery.

The anti-racism action band

After speaking with the school principal and writing a funding application to the local council I was able to contact the Anti Racism Action Band again and invite the group facilitator to come and work with a select group of students in the school. I invited potential participants to write a brief explanation about why they would like to participate in the program and then purposefully selected 15 students from an array of different cultures, including some of the girls who had wanted to be involved. I negotiated with the staff so that the program could take place during class-time and found a room that was more soundproofed than most of the spaces. I then coplanned a series of workshops with the drummer that involved increasingly challenging activities. I also helped to shape his expectations about this particular group of young people, and so it began.

The drummer and I cofacilitated the groups, and once again I was confronted by the fact that my flexible and creative style was not a good match for the other adult. This time we negotiated ahead of time and reached agreements about how we would manage structure and behaviors. He was clear that the students could not be allowed to get out of control and that he demanded respect and control from the beginning so that he could rein things back in if they did get too noisy. Based on the previous session, I conceded that working with larger groups in schools might require a different skill set to that which I had devised for working in small, contained therapy groups. I chose to play a minor role in leadership of this group so that I could maintain my own presence as a nondirective therapeutic presence, and, so that I had the opportunity to learn.

"I didn't see percussion being used as weapons of warfare and conflict. I saw unity and flow."

There were many times during the five workshops where I squirmed at the strict tone of the drummer and thought that a softer tone may have been just as effective. I questioned whether hierarchy was the only way to work with active young men and I had many discussions with the facilitator. He felt that being firm, but not emotional or angry, was entirely appropriate for the development of new skills. He also felt that the cultural backgrounds of the young participants made them more comfortable with the gender- and age-based hierarchy that he required. It was true that the group members learned much more from this drummer than they could have ever learned from me. I will always sacrifice the acquisition of a skill to work with the interpersonal dynamics in a musical process, and this often means that the quality of the musical product is impacted. I did notice looks of rebellion and frustration on the faces of some of the Maori boys at times, but I also saw looks of appreciation and pride when they conquered the skill that had been challenging them. Most importantly, I didn't see percussion being used as weapons of warfare and conflict. I saw unity and flow.

As the weeks passed, I instigated a separate process with some of the group members who were succeeding in the percussion group but struggling the most in school. I selected three boys and three girls to begin teaching the percussion exercises they were learning to some of the younger students in the school. A group of three would enter the classroom and lead the whole group through the exercise they had just learned in the workshop. I modeled these initially and showed them how to generate extension exercises but then quickly moved to the back of the classroom and let the three young people lead through the repetitions. As the weeks passed, I didn't lead the groups at all and instead talked them through different ideas before each class began. I asked them to choose students in the class to come up front with them and show the others what they were doing. I encouraged them to choose girls as well as boys and to make sure they didn't only choose people from their own cultural background. I asked them to improvise new additions to the rhythms they had learned and then to ask some of the class members to try that too. I got to reintroduce the call-and-response exercises I loved so that all group members' voices could be heard.

After some weeks, we decided that the classes would be able to perform at an upcoming concert for the whole school and worked toward perfecting a couple of the routines. When the day came, I was unprepared for the fact that the young leaders were reluctant to stand in front of the whole school and do the actions with the younger children. Although I was aware of this possibility through my training, this particular group of young people had been so comfortable in working with the children until that time, that it caught me by surprise. I talked with the group and did my best to encourage them to lead the young players, with the result that two of the young men were willing to stand near the front. The three younger women could not overcome their fear and were only willing to stand in the back of the group, effectively hiding from view. I was much more prominent than I had planned to be and stood squarely in the middle to conduct the group. It was awkward, but we did it.

"But then an unexpected situation occurred."

The final challenge arose when we turned to the whole school and asked them to join in. This part was too much even for the brave young men on the stage and so I used my own enthusiasm and charm to engage the whole audience in doing the moves. Group members from the workshops were embedded in the crowd, and the percussion games had infiltrated the school over the prior weeks, so I was gradually able to achieve a sufficient amount of participation with the help of those who knew the routines already. But then, another unexpected situation occurred.

A group of the oldest boys had been laughing at the boys on stage throughout the performance. Once again, there was a division along cultural lines, and once again, this led to a slow buildup of energy. As I drew the activity to a close, the volume at the back of the room peaked and I watched with horror as the school principal and a group of other senior teachers marched over to the boys and swiftly ordered them out of the auditorium. They were penalized for their manner of joining in and did not return for the remainder of the performance.

"They established a power hierarchy that seeped through the entire school."

Although there were many aspects of the program that year that were a success, I continued to struggle with this particular dynamic in the school. The zero-tolerance policy was predicated on the desire to keep peace between the cultures, but the implications ran much deeper than managing behavior. They established a power hierarchy that seeped through the entire school and that I was confronted by repeatedly. This was most apparent in the play on the powerful instruments, when instead of providing a way to work with these dynamics, the drums in this context had almost seemed to affirm the fears of the leaders.

I learned that diversity is not always the major challenge to connectedness and inclusion. It can be the adults' responses to the fear of what that diversity might arouse that compounds difficult situations and manifests a tone of enforced power. In that context, my favorite drum-playing activity was a poor match for the needs of the young people. What they needed was something different to what they had already learned. They needed the opportunity to develop new skills and to show leadership by introducing novelty. In many ways, this was achieved, but on reflection, I do feel that it could have been accomplished more readily if I hadn't relied so heavily on my own assumptions from what had worked in the past. Playing music together can transcend difference, but it can also reinforce it. Music is more of a reflection than a game changer, so being open to different possibilities for engaging is as valuable as having a lot of preknowledge about how things might work.

ORCID

Katrina Skewes McFerran ⓘ http://orcid.org/0000-0003-0699-3683

Group Work with Gay Male Teens at the Time of 9/11

Andrew J. Peters

I used to work with lesbian, gay, bisexual, and transgender (LGBT) youth in suburban Long Island, adjacent to New York City. This was well before marriage equality and Bruce Jenner coming out as a transgender woman on prime time TV. Back then, in the 1990s through the early 2000s, the agency I worked for was something of an oasis for LGBT teens in a brutally inhospitable landscape.

Teenagers who had the courage to come out faced hostility on multiple fronts: from their families, their schools, the local churches and synagogues, and not incidentally the media that aired a frightening national dialogue on whether LGBTs should be allowed basic human rights.

I was a young gay man myself, and working intraculturally presented rewards and challenges. I led a group for gay male teens. Besides our age difference (I was in my late twenties at the time), I came from a middle-class, college-educated, politically progressive, and areligious background. The group members were mostly from working-class, politically and religiously conservative families.

Those young men broke me in as a group worker in many essential ways. I was quickly taught that my gayness afforded no special access to under- standing their lives, a lesson that also falls under the category of leaving one's ego at the door. In reaction to my well-intentioned, yet apparently unyielding approach to structure, one group member started calling me, "the Nazi." The nickname caught on with the group, and I came to embrace it with humor.

My planned discussions on topics like coming out and managing painful emotions rarely led to helpful interaction. However, I will always remember a meeting around Halloween when group members wanted to use our weekly time to write horror stories. They read aloud what they wrote at the end of the group, and one story after the other involved me being murdered in some very graphic and gory way. We had a lot of fun at my expense, and beneath the uniquely "boyish" blunt emotional transactions, I sensed that something meaningful was happening.

Around the time of 9/11, we had recently resumed for the school year and I prepared myself to focus on how they were directly and/or indirectly affected by the most devastating act of terrorism that any of us had witnessed. This actually turned out to be an easier topic to broach with the boys than talking about trauma and loss related to being gay. It proved to be a symbolic link to those issues in the long run, but for the purposes of this reflection, I will focus on the surface content of our first discussion.

One of the boys came from a family of generations of New York City police officers, a characteristic of several working-class communities on Long Island. He had a family friend who had died as a first responder to the disaster, and he made curse-filled oaths against "the terrorists." I use quotations because this was during that shell-shocked time when the identities and affiliations of the men who hijacked the planes were unconfirmed but the subject of around-the-clock media speculation. The one constant message in the news was that the terrorists were Muslim and they hated Americans.

Other group members spoke of their belief that more attacks were forthcoming. Some wanted revenge: "to wipe them out before they wipe out us." One young man proudly told a story with a haunting image. His father had recently given him a pick-up truck, and he had tied a picture of a Muslim man on its grill so that everyone would see it when he drove through town. His companions responded favorably.

I chose to give free rein to the discussion. My instincts told me that the foremost concern was allowing the boys to express their fear and anger and even their violent fantasies. They had been robbed of their sense of safety and predictability in the world. The group was their safe place to talk about anything and everything. In their own words, the group was: "a place where we de-stress about the week."

Inside however, I was deeply worried about the discussion. This was a mixed group of boys, primarily White, Catholic, and Jewish with some Black Christian and Hispanic Catholic members. In the absence of Muslim participants, a troubling us versus them mentality had emerged. Some of their language was stridently anti-Muslim, and that image of a photograph strapped to a pick-up truck like a dead deer repulsed me. I was aware of acts of violence against Muslim-owned businesses in recent days. As an antiwar advocate, I was vigilantly attuned to the political rhetoric of the time, which I could feel was leading to a reprisal overseas through which more lives would be lost.

Attending to the group's grieving process needed to be done, but I also wondered if there was an opportunity to broaden their understanding of how defamation affects vulnerable groups. Each of them knew first-hand the injustice and pain of antigay harassment, and they proudly brought to my attention issues of community concern like religious leaders calling gay men "pedophiles" and state ballot initiatives to "defend" marriage from gay people. Could they see the parallel oppression happening to Muslims?

At our next group meeting, I reflected that our last discussion had left me with strong impressions. I was proud of the group for sharing and listening to each other's intense emotional experiences, and notwithstanding my belief that each of them could manage difficult situations, I had left the meeting a little worried about how they were doing during the week. This I recall was received quite profoundly by the young men, who in retrospect I believe had tuned into my unspoken yet still evident disapproval of some of the things that they had said. I then shared that part of my reaction and suggested they might use the group to learn more about the 9/11 attacks and its impact on all of us. I asked if they would be interested in inviting a guest speaker from the Muslim community. The young men thought this was a great idea, and we began to work on questions to ask the speaker.

Now, a brief aside that hammered home the complexity of working with the diversity theme post-9/11. The speaker who was recommended to me was an imam at one of the region's largest mosques. He was a leader in an interfaith initiative to promote tolerance, and he was frequently called upon by the media.

We had a phone call to plan his visit, during which I shared a bit about our discussions in the group. I explained the composition and that the young men might be interested in hearing about gay people growing up in the Muslim faith. The imam's response was that homosexuality was an abomination, and he would need to be clear with them about that point. I told him that he wouldn't be quite right to address the group and thanked him for his time.

A few weeks later, I found a pair of speakers from a grassroots organization working on peace and justice issues from a gay Muslim perspective, and they visited the group. They talked about misconceptions about the Muslim faith and culture, and their efforts to educate beyond and within that community based on their dual and sometimes conflicting identities.

Most of my group members had never had a conversation with a Muslim, and none of them had ever met someone who was Muslim and gay. They were engaged and curious, and their overall impression was admiration and respect. The meeting stretched beyond our 90-minute session, and several group members attended a fundraising event hosted by the organization a few weeks later. From thinking of Muslims as an enemy and a threat, the boys spoke of their appreciation for members of their community who were addressing religious and racial bias. They came to understand their struggles as similar to their own.

Group work around the time of 9/11 helped me to be more aware that being gay put me in the same fleet as my group members but not really the same boat. Age, culture, education, religion, and political affiliation were potential obstacles to understanding what the group needed at the time and finding its way through the diversity theme. Humor, sharing my personal feelings, and introducing diversity helped the group arrive at a new way of looking at the world.

The Watusi Girls: A Legacy of Inspiration

Carol Irizarry

Edie was only age 12 years and had the deepest, most delicate brown eyes that I had ever seen. We sat by the pool on the last day that I would spend with my group, both of us feeling sad and not speaking. I felt tears on my arm and realized that she was crying. Her voice was hesitant and soft but it cut directly into my heart, "Please Carol, just don't forget us."

How could this beautiful young Puerto Rican girl possibly know that during all the years since that moment I could not think of this scene without tears of my own coming to my eyes? Forget her, forget the Watusi girls? Never. They changed me forever.

I had just graduated with my MSW in group work and this this was my first job, my first pay check, my first professional role, my first apartment with friends in New York City, and my first group. Preadolescent girls, from Hispanic and African American backgrounds, asking for help from the settlement house to form a club, which they wanted to call the "Watusi" girls.

They were suspicious when I was "assigned" to them and with good reason. I was green. Naive about New York City life and the issues that these girls encountered on a daily basis. Naïve also about myself and my role as a social group worker. So they went to work on me—imitating my every gesture—my walk, my talk, and my gestures. Mocking Carol was their favorite game. It was humiliating and my anger flared. But then Elba, the president laughed, "It's only a joke," she reassured me. "We do that with everyone."

I needed to respond, but phrases and instructions jumped into my head, "Set boundaries, stay in in control of the interview, this is just a testing phase, focus on the purpose of the group." But how—when? A moment of indecision, a seeming lifetime of hesitation when I felt a crossroads presented itself to me. I took the turn toward humor and instead of reprimand l laughed with them at my silly self. It broke the ice. I trusted Elba, and in return she began to trust me leading the others along that path which of course led back to what they had wanted to do as a group —take trips, go places, have fun, and hang out.

Subway rides were a nightmare as the girls zigzagged around the cars in provocative stances and made rude comments to the other passengers. They were kicked off and I left with them. Then the rebukes started as we walked back in disappointment at the missed trip, "You should have stopped us from being bad on the subway." I had held firm and not taken a behavior-monitoring role and so replied, "You hate people who tell you what to do and I am not a teacher after all. I am a social worker." Confusion emerged, but now they listened seeing me in a different light—something new. This was how talking together began. All summer we walked and talked, and I was able to interject the odd comment about how social workers helped people talk about things that were important to them. Boys were top conversational subjects but school, jobs, parental controls, sex and fear of pregnancies all spilled out.

Their insights into their situations were amazing as were the ideas that emerged in relation to every aspect under consideration. They taught me how they survived with talents such as reading people's real intentions and trusting their own instincts. They showed me their resilience, which was often based on getting up again after being knocked down, literally or symbolically. They revealed to me how such resilience was fostered in their everyday lives. When Naomi's 4-year-old brother tripped and fell down I rushed to help him get up and she stopped me. "He needs to pick himself up," she instructed me, "He needs to learn to be tough."

Above all I discovered how the girls relied on each other for protection and emotional well-being. They displayed a loyalty to their Watusi club that surprised me in its commitment and depth. The fought each other with the same intensity and punished those who did not remain loyal, but they looked out for each other in all situations—another major component of their resilience. And they never tired of teaching me something more about groups and my interactions.

After a clash of wills, I had issued an ultimatum to Cuni, the group clown (and the most accurate at imitating and ridiculing me) that if she disregarded the rule about her young brother one more time she would not be allowed to come on the coveted Coney Island visit. Of course she defied me, and so I forbid her to join us. Maria came to see me alone the next day, pointing out that I had known exactly how Cuni would respond and that I had "set her up" because I didn't like her teasing me and didn't want her included. Another crossroads. Was this true? If so, should I admit it? Should I change my mind? How should I listen to and act on the feedback? I forced myself to look at my motivation and to another way of handling the issue—using Maria's advice and the group members desire to have their friend included. We all went on the trip, and Cuni's behavior was exemplary.

They challenged me to be more real, not to evade, not to hide behind professional language, not to hedge my opinions, and most importantly to integrate my professional and personal roles. They could see through any phony response in 5 seconds flat. Their questions were incessant. "Did I like really them? Would I lend them money? Where did l learn Spanish? Would I take a girl home if her mother died? Did I have a boyfriend? Did I have Puerto Rican friends? Did I have Black friends?" And eventually—best of all, "What did a social worker do anyway?"

I struggled with the meaning behind what they were asking and what they wanted from me. I struggled with answering their concerns while staying within my professional role. Each question challenged me to stay true to my reason for being a social group worker and at the same time to give them an answer that displayed my genuineness, revealing myself as a real person. It was only in answering these questions directly that they began to move into more threatening subjects and raise their encounters around race and pre-judice that they had all experienced. My immediate reactions were always crucial—the pain I felt at their stories—the anger at their hurts. They needed those emotions, and it helped them to view my unadulterated reactions. They also felt conflicted because it was so easy to see "White crackers" as alien and feared, while liking me placed them in peril. The taboo subject of race emerged more frequently, and I needed to help them sort out the conflict rather than suggest solutions, and I needed to avoid being defensive when I was labelled as one of the White oppressors. I kept reminding myself to focus on their needs not mine, on why they had wanted to form a group and what it meant to their lives.

But some topics of conversation led to feelings of self-consciousness accompanied by worries about whether they should be talking about such matter at all, especially with an adult and an outsider. When this happened I reminded the girls of why they had wanted a club in the first place and how my job as a social worker was to help them with everything they wanted to do together, including talking about things that were tough or unusual. This usually provided enough justification for delving into subjects which raised anxiety.

As for the individual Watusi girls, I stood in awe of their strength and their ability to find ways to live creative lives within their environment. I latched on this resilience and tried to contribute to its power, to their understanding of each other and their engagement in the world around them. They were powerful girls —rich in character, energy, humor, and resolve. I shared in their adventures and challenges. And I fell in love with them.

I learned social work. I learned group work. I learned about myself, and I gave myself to these girls with whom I walked the streets of New York. These were the same girls who teased me mercilessly until the day I left, who cried on my shoulder about family problems and fights with friends, who called me "White cracker," and then threw their arms around me when I came back from a holiday. They were the same girls who all slept touching me, with every single girl holding onto a part of me when we camped on Bear Mountain and slept outside. Tough on the streets of East Harlem but afraid of a dark night without streetlights.

I see their faces clearly and vividly. Edie, Elba, Cuni, Maria, Norma, Shirley, Brenda, Naomi, and Miranda. I mix up their real names with the code names that I gave them in writing and talking about them over the decades, but their faces remain young, vibrant, and distinct before me now—years after they would have grown to be mothers and grandmothers.

"No Edie," I replied, "I will never forget you." And I never have. You showed me strength and vulnerability—and gave me trust and affection. You came with the other girls to my wedding. Still a group but with your new worker and I saw your beaming faces as a precious part of that celebration—a gift of lasting influence, frozen in the picture frames.

You and your friends molded me and sculptured me into the social worker that I became and remained. It was through working with you and the other Watusi girls that the words I had read in textbooks transformed in actions in the real world. And I learned that all the social work theories, skills, techniques, ideas, and insights, however relevant, must be carried out through a genuineness of self and a feeling of true affection. The most challenging skill of all is to be real and professional at the same time and to hold that delicate balance.

I close my eyes and I can feel again Edie's tears on my arm as she sits by the pool. I wish I could tell her and the other Watusi girls of their effect on my development and my gratitude for the social group work they taught me. "No Edie I have never forgotten you and I never will."

Creating Space for LGBTQ Youths to Guide the Group

Karen Myers

6:50 p.m. 6:55 p.m. 6:57 p.m.
The group time is set for 7–8:30 p.m.
 No one is early.
 At 7 the first member
 Saunters through the door.
 "Is this where the LGB-whatever group is meeting?"
 "It is," I reply, and
 "Welcome."
 We are quickly joined by others.
 As members go around the circle and introduce themselves -
 Name, pronoun, why they've come.
 We are rich in diversity.
 An LGBTQ group for youth was advertised
 And it is quickly apparent that involves an intersection
 Of many different lines.
 Yet a common theme emerges quickly.
 They come hungry for a sense of belonging
 And a desire to be accepted and understood
 For who they are.
 Ground rules involving respect are laid.
 Then the floodgates open as
 Heart-breaking stories of ostracism, bullying, and abuse
 Are shared again and again.
 Many are on the streets.
 Some are living with a friend.
 A few are in foster care.
 Two are at home
 But neither knows for how much longer.
 School is a battleground.
 They report feeling lucky
 If they are simply called names.
 When one member sought help from a school administrator
 He was told playing a sport might help him fit in better

Even after he reported that the locker room during
Physical education was when he was routinely harassed
By his peers.
They are damned in church
And shunned by their family members.
They lose friends and safety.
These young people have every reason to be hardened
And closed off
And unwilling to risk
Again
But in that very first meeting
They begin to support each other
And offer what they have
To the group process.
In the following weeks
I am humbled and amazed
Again and again.
I am ready with my group work knowledge
Theories
Facilitation techniques and
Topics for discussion.
A new group member
Who I fear may not fit in is readily absorbed
Just as she is.
When one of the two members still living at home
Gets kicked out by his pastor father
With only the clothes he is wearing
There is no shortage of offerings made to him
By those who have so little themselves.
My role is often limited
Once the group gets going because
They ask the questions
They've wanted to answer themselves.
They offer the resources
They've learned to count on for survival.
They draw quieter members out.
They orient new members as they come in.
They listen without judgment.
They laugh without mocking.
They cry without pitying.
No one tries to change anyone.
Just showing up to the group
Is an act of courage

But these young people
Offer each other
What they have not been given themselves
Dignity
Respect
And a place to belong.
All I have to do is provide them space
Freedom
And a willingness to listen.

I felt a connection with group members before I even met them. It was the late 1990s and the group evoked in me my own struggle with self-identity, growing up as a teenager in the 1980s and coming out to myself as a lesbian. My family was religious, and I knew intimately the fear, the worry, the suffocation, and the self-doubt that were my constant companions in my teenage years. Thankfully I also remembered how desperate I was for someone to listen and accept me for who I was. I had gone through my process then. Now, 10 years later, this was their process.

I had envisioned myself as a group worker. I had ideas about how to foster group cohesion and guide the development of the group. I thought I had so much to offer this group now that I was out and comfortable with myself. I was aware that I needed to resist the desire to unilaterally swoop in to provide the support, advice, and counsel I had wanted at their age. I didn't want to minimize their capacities or ability to offer mutual aid. They were told by far too many adults that they did not know themselves, were making poor choices, were aberrant, and could not be trusted.

Shame and guilt

Many of the group members reported struggling with shame and guilt. They wondered if they were the cause of their problems as they had been told. As they sat and listened to similar experiences shared by their fellow group members they began to recognize and understand how societal structures contributed to their being marginalized and oppressed. Their families, schools, and churches were trying to make them fit into a certain mold. What they knew was that being lesbian, gay, bisexual, transgender, queer (LGBTQ) did not fit that mold. It was the very same mold I had found hard to fit in to 10 years prior and the same mold many are struggling to fit now almost 20 years later. The group realized that they were all in the same boat. The empathy and support that each one expressed extended, full circle, to themselves.

There was a freedom in the group that few had experienced before. Taboo subjects that they were hesitant to bring up in other settings were openly discussed in the group. One week safe-sex practices were discussed. Although many of them had participated in some form of sex education in their health and physical education classes, few had heard of dental dams or safe-sex practices for anal sex. One group discussion revolved around hormone therapy and ways to minimize bodily parts that betrayed. Wearing tight sports bras and sometimes additional binding allowed several of the young women to minimize the appearance of their breasts. Some of the young men discussed ways to hide the appearance of their external genitals. The group became especially lively as members laughed about what parts they would be willing to readily trade.

Transformation and visibility

Several group members visibly changed as they came to group week after week, becoming comfortable enough to put on the clothes and accessories that felt most representative of their true selves. A slight young man, who identified as gay to the group, began to wear make-up, press on nails, and wigs, often transforming in the bathroom right before group started. He was soon joined by another group member and the two came into group sharing and comparing their finds of the week. An unknowing older sister was a frequent supplier and was thanked in absentia during group for being an avid if unorganized collector of her younger brother's fantasies so that he could raid her room without detection. It was prayer-like when he closed his glittered eyelids and offered, "Thank you, Big Sis, for your cluttered room full of glamour for me." "Thank you and amen from me," followed his friend. "I need a big brother," added one of the young women who had begun binding her breasts after she shaved part of her head.

I was amazed by the resourcefulness of group members. They were able to aid each other in ways I could not have imagined. Between them, they knew most of the 24-hour restaurants and bars where gay-friendly proprietors did not ask questions if a young person needed a place to be. One Starbucks manager was even known to graciously provide a free hot drink to soothe an aching heart. Although I had been terrified about coming out to my family when I was their age, I did not think I would end up homeless, like so many of the group had. Quite a few of the young men who had been kicked out of their homes talked openly with each other about how to turn tricks safely. They spoke of wealthy, discrete businessmen who were kind and willing to pay well for secrecy. It was unsettling to learn that often life on the streets was considered as safe if not safer than living in a home, especially if the home was one of the notorious group homes for teenagers in foster care. The unspoken rules in those places were far more important to learn than the posted house rules. Survival for LGBTQ youth was dependent on knowing them. I had no idea.

One of the more masculine young women in the group described how it was much safer to be thought of as "crazy" than simply "butch" in the group home where she lived. She had been targeted and harassed until she noticed how everyone steered a clear path around another young woman who often sat mumbling to herself or shouting threats to no one in particular. She adopted similar mannerisms to protect herself. Other group members shared how they aligned with group home staff by doing favors for them as a way to gain some protection.

Visibility was desired and feared. Hoodies on the street could cover a short haircut or a face longing for false eyelashes and bright red lipstick. In group, tattered pictures of cherished moments of freedom were pulled out of baggy pockets and passed around. One group member shaved the bottom part of her head but left long hair on top to cover it up when needed. She shared pictures of herself with the long hair pulled back and wished she "could shave it all off."

Another group member shared a picture everyone thought was his sister until he proudly said the picture was of him. "Pretty" morphed from a threat to a compliment simply because the place was safe. "You're too damn pretty to be a boy" was a high compliment in this group, whereas it was cause for fear on a deserted subway ride. Invisibility was valued there. "Pull your hood up, put headphones on, and slouch in your seat like you asleep," were instructions for a new group member who was being harassed on his subway rides to school.

> Yeah, but don't listen to anything so you always know what's going on around you. Sometimes if I hear shit starting, I act like it's my stop so I can get off and get on the next train. I'd rather be late than beat.

"Choose crowded cars if you can and sit near anyone with young children or old people cause they don't mess with you."

Pride and public exposure

When they decided as a group they wanted to walk in the upcoming gay pride parade, I stepped back as they took ownership of the preparations. They strategized about different ways to protect members who did not want to be seen, at the same time they celebrated their fellow members who were eager to be visible. Brightly colored signs covered in rainbows and pink triangles were made to celebrate symbols of solidarity while also providing a shield for those who wanted one. Large rainbow flags could be waved or used as a shroud. What might have appeared to be a random assortment of young people on the day of the parade was as carefully choreographed as a ballet. "I'll walk here with the end of our banner because I want everyone to see these fabulous stilettos." "Girl, they won't see anyone else with you sashaying like that," "If I hold this sign, I can hide behind it if I see someone I don't want to see me," and "You can even wear a wig and some sunglasses if you want more protection."

Fear, solidarity, and empowerment

When Matthew Shepard was beaten and left to die in a rural area of Wyoming, the group mourned and memorialized his death with artwork and poetry. Matthew was age 21 years at the time of his murder in October 1998 in Laramie, Wyoming. He was beaten, tortured, and left to die by two young men who targeted him due to his sexual orientation. This was an experience that many in the group feared, especially those surviving on the streets because they needed the money they earned by getting into cars with men they often did not know. Matthew's murder reinforced the risks they knew they were taking.

During the group meeting in which they shared their creations, I asked if they would like me to explore the possibility of exhibiting their artwork and poetry publicly, allowing any group member to display his or her work anonymously or opt out entirely. They uniformly did not want Matthew's death to be forgotten, and every member ended up participating to the extent he or she felt comfortable. All of them exhibited their work, but some chose not to put their names on it. Their bravery in the face of a tragedy that encompassed some of their own daily risks and greatest fears was yet another example of their resiliency. They again negotiated appearing in a public space by protecting one another. As they prepared for the exhibit, a group member wrote down the names of those who wanted their works identified and those who did not. As she wrote, she commented that she was willing to do either if not identifying her work was needed so there were enough anonymous pieces or identifying her work so there was more solidarity and support for those who did. Others agreed they were willing to do whatever the group needed most.

The group's exhibit was displayed for a month on the walls in one of the gathering spaces of the organization where the group met. There were realistic paintings depicting the desolation of the field and the fence where Matthew was tied along with abstract pieces that seemed to howl with pain and isolation. One young woman framed her poem with raffia to look like field grasses and interspersed them with red yarn that flowed off the bottom of the frame to pool on the floor like blood. The group talked about the conversations they overheard as well as ones they participated in. They were heartened by the support they felt from many and devastated by comments that suggested Matthew "deserved what happened to him." Although expressed in different ways, group members were united in their collective voice of support and sorrow for Matthew through the exhibit. Even after the exhibit ended, the group's cohesiveness and protectiveness towards each other was buoyed by the experience. There were more numbers exchanged and more contacts outside of group to check on each other.

Lessons learned

Despite recent progress in the legal landscape regarding LGBTQ equality, legislation does not ensure safety for young people coming out today. Sadly, the voices I hear in LGBTQ groups in 2015 are echoes of the voices of the young people written about in this article. They often share similar experiences of oppression and marginalization as they attempt to find acceptance and belonging in their families, churches, and schools.

A lesson learned for me is that the road to oppression may be paved with good intentions and that I need to know when to get out of the way to promote group autonomy. The LGBTQ youths in this group needed space for their own agency to be recognized. This required me, the group worker, to gradually reduce my centrality and turn control over to the group. I cooperated with their efforts by valuing and supporting their self-direction, as opposed to being one more adult hell-bent on making them conform to my ideas of what the group needed based on my own coming out experience. All they needed was the room to breathe and safe space.

From Profiled to Praiseworthy to Proud

Andrew Malekoff

In 2008 I joined together with a group of community advocates to conduct an action research study that we had hoped might offer some insight into the concerns and needs of immigrant youth and families living in Nassau County, New York. According to the U.S. Census Bureau, this suburb of New York City then has a population of 1,339,552 of which nearly 20% of the residents are foreign born and 25% speak languages other than English at home (2011).

The survey results offered insight into the felt needs of immigrant youth, their experiences in accessing services, and their perceptions of the gaps in existing services. The survey also included space for the youth's voices with respect to the impact of immigration status on their daily life that included academic performance, fear of family deportation, and lack of access to healthcare.

At the same time that the action research project was in development, the dominating national news story, with its local origin, was the killing of Ecuadorean immigrant Marcello Lucero. The deadly and unprovoked assault, the result of a bias attack by a group of seven Long Island high school students, sent a sobering message to all those involved with teenagers on Long Island. Although cries of "hate crime" rang out, this horrific event was a reminder that diversity is an issue for every adolescent.

Two goals of the action research were raising consciousness and stimulating interaction. To that end, when the survey was completed, we organized an intergenerational, cross-cultural forum "Understanding the Concerns and Needs of Immigrant Youth in Nassau County, New York."

The participating teens and adults of different ethnic backgrounds, including immigrants from multiple communities, listened to a summary of the survey results and commented on relevance between the findings and their own lives. Prominent themes in the discussion included diversity, stereotypes and oppression, cultural self-awareness, and understanding of and respect for cultural differences.

Several adult participants who immigrated to the United States shared their struggles. One Spanish speaker expressed (through a translator) her difficulties managing daily life without mastering the English language. Others spoke of being victims of discrimination. Most dramatic was one young teenage boy who revealed a painful truth to the group.

The forum was organized in a combination large- and small-group format designed to build trust and intimacy, as a number of the issues hit close to home for the participants. During one segment when all 35 of us were seated together in a large circle, I scanned the room and my eyes were drawn to 13-year-old Muhammad who was listening intently to the others telling personal stories about leaving their homelands and struggling to fit in after arriving in the United States. In time, as the forum's facilitator, I turned to the boy and said, "Muhammad, it looks to me like you might have something to share with the group."

Muhammad revealed, with a trembling voice, that there were kids in school who taunted him. "They've been calling me "terrorist" for years because of my name." *Muhammad* is an Arabic name that means *praiseworthy*. But, instead of him feeling proud, Muhammad felt like an outcast.

Muhammad sat slumped in his chair and spoke softly and guardedly, but clearly and eloquently; and he was heard. By the end of the day he had received so much support from the group for having the courage to address a taboo subject that he was beaming.

Muhammad's was a story that I had heard other versions of before. As I recall, so fearful was one Muslim mother who lived in the same community, at the center of which is a prominent mosque, that she dyed her children's hair a lighter color to prevent them, as she said, from being profiled as "kin of terrorists."

During lunch break I approached Muhammad and asked him how he was doing. He said, "Everybody is telling me that I talked so good. I didn't know that I could talk so good. Nobody ever told me that before." Muhammad left the meeting feeling praiseworthy, a feeling befitting his name, a name that he was given at birth that he should feel proud to have.

As we remember all those who were lost to acts of terror throughout the world, we should not lose sight of the fact that profiling people of Middle-Eastern descent as terrorists or as sympathizers must be confronted in our groups.

More than 1,000 youths responded to the action research survey that was the impetus for the intergenerational forum. Although it was in the forum and not in the survey that the theme of profiling related to terrorism emerged, the survey generated responses about a multitude of other fears experienced by young people for whom immigration was central to their lives.

They included fear regarding deportation and experiencing discrimination. As one survey respondent wrote, "The problem with immigration is sometimes we have to hide like we are bad persons." This was a feeling that Muhammad, for different reasons, knew very well.

The group forum was an activity that was used to activate interaction among diverse groups of young and older people. By taking a risk to contribute to the dialogue and be heard, Muhammad experienced personal change—a new confidence and acceptance among others who also shared painful stories of trying to fit in and knowing the pain of feeling, sometimes, like they had to hide.

In this group, many people's eyes were opened by simply listening to the painful account of a profiled 13-year-old boy who took the risk to tell his story.

References

U.S. Census Bureau. (2011). *State and county quickfacts: Nassau County, NY.* Retrieved from http://quickfacts.census.gov/qfd/states/36/36059.html

AGING

"The closest thing to being cared for is to care for someone else."
Carson McCullers

A Different Kind of Sorority

Charlene Lane

Sometimes group work happens in unusual places and under unconventional circumstances, as my story about an encounter with a group of women who were marginalized and disenfranchised and were seeking some catharsis illustrates. The group took place at an all-female correctional facility in central Pennsylvania where female inmates age 55 years and older participated in an impromptu group, following a research study that my colleague and I conducted.

The initial goal of the visit was to administer quantitative and qualitative surveys to obtain information about the lived experiences of these women who are not eligible for parole and aging in the penal community. However, what transpired once the data was collected was spontaneous, unrehearsed, and revealing.

When the data collection was complete the women in the group requested a meeting to debrief. Even though the protocol of the interview clearly stipulated that inmates will be afforded the opportunity to communicate with the Department of Corrections' therapist if needed; they requested to "speak with" my colleague (not a clinically trained professional) and me.

Their request set off a plethora of ethical whistles in me. There were pros and cons, I thought. Do I have permission to do this? I am a trained and licensed clinician, but I was working at the facility in my capacity as an educator and researcher, not therapist. Other ethical issues came to mind such as the safety of the inmates. For example, I wondered, what if they were to express negative thoughts and feelings about the facility's employees, some of whom might be in the room. And, I thought about what our moral obligation to the women was, especially because we would most likely never see them again or have an opportunity to follow up with any of their concerns.

On the pro side of the equation, I thought about the benefits of brief therapeutic interventions. And, so, I sought and obtained verbal permission from the prison warden to conduct a 50-minute support/debriefing group at the all-female correctional facility.

The group participants were from diverse ethnic, racial, socioeconomic, and educational backgrounds. They ranged from gang members to professional people.

The inmate who requested the meeting was clearly the leader. She was most vocal and encouraged her peers to express themselves because according to her, "We have someone from the outside who is willing to listen." Initially, there was a brief period of uncertainty and ambivalence among the group members. There was some anxiety, especially because there were correction facility employees in the room. Within a short time, however, members and facilitators became more comfortable as the pace and level of dialogue and interaction picked up. Each member expressed her feelings and concerns as they pertained to growing old as women and to the unique challenges of growing old behind bars with no hope of being released.

Even though the participants in this group came from many walks of life there was one unifying theme—they were all found guilty of a crime that resulted in them being imprisoned without the possibility of parole.

One inmate shared that she used to be a social worker and admired the work that my colleague and I were doing. She was very articulate and struck a chord in me. I wondered to myself, what could this well-educated, poised, well-spoken woman have possibly done to end up in prison? What I learned later was that the former social worker (along with her daughter) was a victim of domestic violence. Consequently, she murdered the perpetrator. I also learned that this was a similar scenario for others in the group.

Many participants disclosed their discontent with the health care they were receiving, stating that there was a long waiting period to see a physician. They said that they were not heard when they expressed physical complaints.

The older inmates shared feelings about their mortality and provided valuable advice to the younger ones. Even though there was some trepidation about dying in prison and ultimately being forgotten, the inmates expressed value in the prison hospice program. This program permits healthy inmates to care for those with terminal illnesses. This provided a sense of comfort for those who feared dying alone.

They could see the reciprocity inherent in caring for others and then having someone care for them if they became ill. The oldest member of the group, who was in her late eighties, disclosed that she was confident that her "younger" cell mate would "look out" for her when her time came. It is important to note that the other members of the group expressed their desire to care for the sick and dying among them.

I would be remiss not to mention the nonverbal yet very present factor in the group that could have inhibited the fluidity of the group process. Throughout the meeting there was a corrections officer and several other Department of Corrections officials in the room. Even though they were not active participants there were subtle nonverbal cues, such as facial grimaces, that could have influenced what the inmates disclosed. Nevertheless, this group of incarcerated women, age 55 to 80, took a leap of faith. The result was a healthy, cathartic experience.

Although only a one-time brief group, a feeling of family emerged. Just as in group therapy with a kinship group, this group of inmates had their own "language" and unique manner of interacting with one another. Clearly this "sorority" had a relationship outside the brief group experience. There were able-bodied inmates who were committed to transporting their wheel chair–bound peers. There were others who felt compelled to clarify what some of their fellow inmates were struggling to express.

For example, there was one inmate who wanted my colleague and me to guarantee changes as it pertained to the wait time to see a physician. Another inmate quickly clarified that that was not our role and function. I felt like an outsider, grappling with quickly trying to understand the unspoken language among members of this group.

In addition to a sense of familial cohesion, there was a clear sense of respect among the members who allowed one another the space to share their concerns and, at times, provided comfort to one another. For example, one group member shared, after another revealed she was a grandmother, "I am a grandmother too and I miss having the opportunity to see my grandchildren grow."

Or there was the inmate who provided concrete advice to her peer who stated that because she is severely arthritic; climbing to her upper bunk bed was becoming quite challenging.

Another member openly shared her phobia of heights and, as the result of not being assigned an upper bunk, she went on to disclose that she is grateful for the mental health care she is now receiving. According to her "there was something always not right with me but no one could tell me what it was." This group member-inmate was alluding to her grappling with undiagnosed psychiatric issues prior to incarceration.

It was important that this forgotten population was afforded the opportunity to have this group experience. After about 50 minutes, the corrections officer signaled to my colleague and me that we had to start wrapping things up. The inmates thanked us for taking the time to hear their concerns. I felt a legitimate sense of gratitude. I was sure to assure them that my colleague and I would pass on their concerns to the "powers that be" but there is no promise of immediate change.

The inmates were encouraged to support each other and "look out" for each other. I left the group with the echo of one of my heartfelt beliefs: Family is not necessarily people you are related to by blood, but people who are good to you and good for you.

I left the prison that day with mixed emotions, being grateful for the path my own life has taken, being appreciative of freedom and being able to go home to my family. Then there was a sense of deep sadness. I was saddened by the fact that without some opportunity and support, an individual's life can be forever altered. Stepping away from the group, I was also left with the thought that there is so much pain in the world. This saddened me further.

The inmates in this group taught me more than they will ever know. Despite the cards dealt to them and their life sentences, the inmates were resilient women, mothers, grandmothers, sisters and friends. They were articulate advocates who respected, cherished and loved the FAMILY they had become.

Incarcerated individuals age 55 and older are a steadily increasing population that includes significant numbers of inmates who are in prison for life as the result of crimes committed in their youth. It is imperative that this vulnerable population is not forgotten.

Group work in prison can offer otherwise voiceless older adults who are incarcerated to find some catharsis in a safe, holding environment and provide them with an opportunity to express many heartfelt fears and concerns that might otherwise go overlooked or unheard.

Lessons Learned from Ballroom Dancing with Older Adults

Ann M. Rodio and Alexandria Holmes

Introduction

During the spring of 2015, we were two MSW students who collaborated on a pilot program for the benefit of older adults. We began with the usual literature review for the purpose of defining the target population, their specific needs, and evidence-based research that identified effective interventions for the elderly population. We learned that the aging of the baby boomer generation, advances in medicine, and increasing racial and ethnic diversity are factors that demand that more emphasis be placed on the development of creative, preventive approaches to improve physical, mental, and emotional health conditions for a diverse population of aging Americans. After researching a broad range of issues and interventions for older adults, we chose to utilize ballroom dance as a psychosocial intervention for older adults.

Ballroom dance as a psychosocial intervention

We initially determined that that the main research question for the study would be whether participation in a ballroom dance group would help older adults to master unresolved ego conflicts as described by Erik Erikson's eight stages (Erikson & Erikson, 1997), thereby preparing them for a more peaceful transcendence during their final years of life. To examine this hypothesis, Ann created a survey instrument comprising questions intended to measure each participant's self-rated level of Erikson's eight syntonic qualities: trust, autonomy (independence), initiative (creativity), industry (competence), identity (sense of self), intimacy, generativity (accomplishment), and integrity (fulfillment). We selected an assisted living facility to participate in a study, obtained Institutional Review Board approval, and prepared to visit the assisted living facility to recruit participants.

Research method and adaptations

We learned throughout our MSW program that quantitative instruments have numerous benefits including ease of use and generalizability. As such,

Color versions of one or more of the figures in the article can be found online at www.tandfonline.com/wswg

we planned to conduct a pretest/posttest study designed to measure the degree to which participation in a ballroom dance event changed the self-rated level of Erikson's eight syntonic qualities (Erikson & Erikson, 1997). However, we quickly discovered that the elderly population at the assisted living facility presented a unique set of circumstances that required us to alter the research question and the method of inquiry. Several of the residents of this particular assisted living facility were "memory-care patients," meaning they had some measure of memory impairment such as dementia or Alzheimer's disease. The first research obstacle we faced was how to obtain informed consent from the residents who would be participating in or observing the dance. None of the residents who was identified by facility staff as potential dancers had the ability to sign their own informed consent forms. Thankfully, the director of nursing and the activity coordinator offered to contact the family members on our behalf, either by phone or when they came to visit their family member. This brings up an important aspect of how to successfully work with this population. We had developed a relationship with the staff by visiting the facility several times just to socialize with the residents and participate in facility activities. This relationship brought the staff into the study as invested participants who were willing to support the project in any way they could.

Once the plan for obtaining consent forms was in place, we visited the facility to conduct the pretests utilizing the survey instrument. However with the first resident, it was quickly discovered that quantitative methods were not going to be feasible with this population. Furthermore, it became apparent that quantitative methods would not do an effective job of capturing the vast amount of wisdom, knowledge, and stories that these residents had to offer. With this realization, we quickly improvised by using the instrument as a general guide for conducting semistructured qualitative interviews. The residents and we benefited greatly from this method adaptation that allowed participants the opportunity to share their stories openly and at their own pace. Through these stories, we gained insight into the importance of dance in the lives of the facility residents while they were growing up.

The dance

The dance (Figure 1) was held on a Saturday afternoon under the guidance of the same professional dance organization that had conducted the beginner's dance classes at the university. All of the assisted living residents who were physically capable of leaving their room attended the dance. A total of six residents actually participated by dancing. One of residents who danced the entire time was heard to say, "Today was the best day!" Another resident dancer said that she had gone dancing a lot with her sister while growing up but that it had been so long since she danced. She said, "I really just wanted

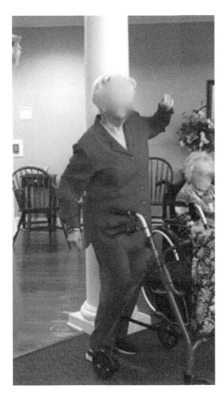

Figure 1. Her eyes sparkled while she reminisced about previous Valentine's Day dances.

to see if I still could. And I did!" One resident, who was confined to a wheelchair and unable to communicate verbally due to severe dementia, was observed keeping rhythm to the music by gently tapping her fingertips together throughout the entire event. Everyone involved considered the dance (Figure 2) to be a huge success with lots of fun, food, music, conversation, and laughter enjoyed by all of the residents and the facility care staff.

During the two weekends that immediately followed the dance, we opted again to forgo use of the survey and posed open-ended questions to the same residents who had participated in the predance interviews. Residents were asked about their experiences either dancing or observing the other residents who danced. Once again, we were pleasantly surprised by the wisdom and depth of meaning found in the responses that were provided. One frequent response given was commentary about one of the residents in memory care who danced to every song that was played. As many of the residents noted, this particular resident often forgets who and where she is, but during the dance she was improvising and dancing as her procedural memory overcame her memory impairment. We learned that this particular resident had been a ballerina and even owned her own dance studio in her younger days. All of

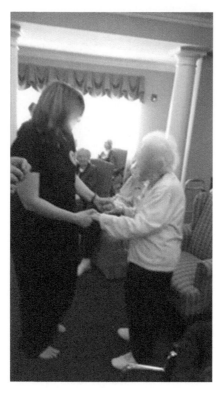

Figure 2. She was curious and determined to know if she could still dance.

the residents who discussed observing her noted how great it was to see her enjoying herself and how her body remembered how to dance even if her brain had lost many of her memories.

One of the residents who participated in the dance event illustrated the positive psychosocial impact of dancing as she underwent a transformation from a quiet, shy, reserved lady to the belle of the ball. During the predance interview, she told us about how she grew up in Hattiesburg. She said there used to be many more soldiers stationed at her hometown military base when she was younger, and that she and "the girls" would go dance with the soldiers "because the soldiers enjoyed it so much." She also said with a schoolgirl giggle that "we just danced though. We never went anywhere with the soldiers; we just went to dance. We would go all the time and it was so much fun." She explained how dances were a big part of her social life at that time. During the dance, she was hesitant at first but agreed to dance after receiving some encouragement from the researchers and the facility staff. She found a dance partner and proceeded to dance to every song that was played. Several of the facility care staff members expressed their surprise at seeing this shy, quiet lady dancing with statements such as, "I cannot believe she is dancing. She is usually so shy. I just cannot believe it!" After the

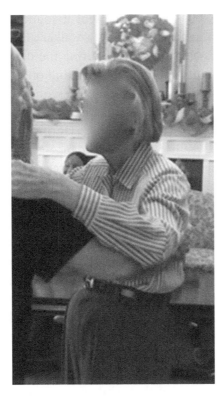

Figure 3. Normally quiet and reserved, she danced to every song and stated that dancing was "freeing."

dance, the resident said that she had a wonderful time and that the dance had brought back fun memories. She said that dancing was "freeing," and she hoped that another dance could be held again soon (Figure 3).

Immediately following the dance, this resident informed us that she found the dance to be "stimulating" and "good for everyone." She talked about how she is still able to drive and completely care for herself but chooses to live in the facility because she does not want to be a burden to her family. She said that she often gets bored in the facility and feels "confined" because she is able to do more physically than what the facility lifestyle allows. She said that she felt less confined during the dance and that the event was a "good change of pace" for all of the residents. She said that because her husband never wanted to dance, she had not danced since her younger days with the soldiers at her hometown military base. She said she "loves being able to do it again."

One particular resident personified the positive impact that just observing dance can have on an older adult. She was a feisty lady who was not particularly interested in speaking to us prior to the dance. When she was introduced to us by the director of nursing and asked if she would be willing to talk for a few minutes, she replied, "Well, okay. I guess it would be alright to talk a minute. Let's just get this over with." She informed everyone that she would not be dancing, but that she thought it sounded like a good idea for "the others." She explained that she uses a walker all of the time and would not be interested in dancing. However, during the dance, the same lady was observed smiling, laughing, and tapping her hand on her leg in rhythm to the music. She was heard to comment that everyone who was dancing was "brave" and that she "was proud of them." When asked if she was enjoying herself she replied, "Oh yes. This is lovely." During the follow-up interview, she explained that she was not allowed to dance growing up because "I was Baptist, you know." She said that she did wish her daughter had known about the dance so that she could have come to watch with her. When asked if she thought additional dances would be a good idea, she replied, "Yes, yes that would be nice. I would tell my daughter next time." When asked whether she thought others enjoyed the dance, she emphatically said, "Well I think so. I really think they did, but I cannot speak for everyone." When asked to explain why she thought the others enjoyed the dance, she replied, "Why? Well, they just did!" with an attitude and look that expressed how obvious it was to everyone that all participants enjoyed themselves and what a silly question it was to ask why. Before the postdance interview was concluded, this feisty lady asked at least three times, "When did you say you might come again?" She said that she wanted to be sure to tell her daughter to come the next time. She also commented that while she was not allowed to dance as a young girl, she had always encouraged her daughter to dance as a form of personal expression. These are just a few examples of the residents we were able to interact with during this project and their incredible responses we witnessed as a result of the dance event and our surrounding visits.

Lessons learned

With any study population, but particularly the elderly population, building relationships is an important part of conducting research. Without the relationship, in-depth, meaningful information is less likely to come from the research. As such, the first lesson learned served to reinforce the fundamental social work core value of the importance of human relationships and the concept of client-centered interaction. The initial selection of a structured survey intended to measure the relative change in abstract, psychosocial qualities in the older adult population was inappropriate for what this population had to offer. The residents were interested in sharing their stories at their own pace, and they only did so once they became comfortable with who the researchers were and why they were there. The longer we were willing to sit and listen, the more rich and colorful their stories became, showing the depth of wisdom contained within each resident, unique to their own personal histories.

The importance of building relationships may even be more critical to successful work with this population than others. Without the initial visitations and relationship building, the dance event may not have even occurred. During the predance interviews, residents were polite and would answer direct questions, but the answers would be surface level and conversations were kept at a minimum. However, during the dance and postdance interviews, residents were much more open to conversation and willing to spend a few hours discussing dancing, music, relationships, and significant life events. Furthermore, the interactions among the residents changed over the course of the project. During initial visits, residents were not only reserved from researchers, but many were disengaged from one another. For example, in one baking activity we attended, none of the residents interacted with one another but only interacted with the staff member leading the activity upon being prompted. A stark contrast was found during the dancing event, during which residents were actively engaged with those around them, including the staff and other residents. The power of the group was evident during the event at which time the residents were participating and engaged as a member of the group as a whole; we observed a sense of "oneness."

The second lesson learned was the power of procedural memory. Much research has been published to support the idea that physical activity can help older adults to maintain and improve their quality of life. We saw this concept in action through the phenomenon of procedural memory and the use of reminiscence in story-telling. In our review of the literature, we had learned through procedural memory, motor skill memories are relatively unaffected by the aging process and that new ones can be learned and improved at any age (Seidler, 2007; Smith et al., 2005). We witnessed this phenomenon while observing fairly residents who were immobile and memory affected dance with the ease of an amateur ballroom dancer. Through the dance, residents were allowed to either experience the thrill of this type of physical activity or witness their fellow residents enjoy dancing. As a result, they became more likely to open up and reminisce about their younger days. The music and movement allowed older adults to reconnect with their memories and bring them into the present. This reconnection demonstrated by participants during the dance is consistent with studies that report how reminiscence encourages older adults to share their histories with one another to find common ground, and increases a sense of belonging (Hamill, Smith, & Rohricht, 2011).

Lastly, an important lesson learned through this experience was how valuable information can be gained even when a study fails to prove an initial hypothesis. The original research question involving Erikson's syntonic ego qualities (Erikson & Erikson, 1997) was too abstract to lend itself to being captured quantitatively with the elderly population. Regardless and perhaps because of this obstacle, we gained significant experience in conducting research, remaining flexible, and learning how to build relationships with the elderly population.

Concluding personal reflections

Throughout this process, we were reminded of the importance of building relationships and starting where the client is, particularly for research with groups different from ourselves. The population we worked with does not easily open up and completing quantitative surveys does not interest them. They desire relationships and a sense of community which qualitative research can offer. In our work with this group, the "client" wanted to share an afternoon with us, learning from one another and simply fellowshipping. By following our instinct and social work values, we were able to start where this particular population was coming from and in return gained enormous insight into how to work with this population. It is our hope that by sharing our experience, we can help other social workers to learn from our research efforts as they expand their knowledge and design creative interventions for improving the quality of life for our cherished elderly population.

References

Erikson, E. & Erikson, J. (1997). *The life cycle completed: Extended version*. London, UK: W. W. Norton.

Hamill, M., Smith, L., & Rohricht, F. (2012). Dancing down memory lane: Circle dancing as a psychotherapeutic intervention in dementia—A pilot study. *Dementia, 11*(6), 709–724. doi:10.1177/1471301211420509

Seidler, R. D. (2007). Older adults can learn to learn new motor skills. *Behavioural Brain Research, 183*(1), 118–122. doi:10.1016/j.bbr.2007.05.024

Smith, C., Walton, A., Loveland, A., Umberger, G., Kryscio, R., & Gash, D. M. (2005). Memories that last in old age: Motor skill learning and memory preservation. *Neurobiology of Aging, 26*(6), 883–890. doi:10.1016/j.neurobiolaging.2004.08.014

FROM MEDICAL MODEL TO SOCIAL MODEL

"We need to treat illnesses above
the neck the same as we treat
illnesses below the neck."

Unknown

"Oh, Don't Get Your Hopes up about That. He'll Never Be the Same"

Joseph Walsh

I once had a graduate social work student who was as sensitive to human diversity as anyone I've ever known. Paradoxically, she objected whenever I introduced a topic in class on a specific type of diverse population. "It's artificial to talk about diversity in these ways," she'd say. "All of us are diverse, because we're unique human beings." Her sentiment had a lasting effect on me. I began to look at all my clients as diverse compared to me (a White male), even when they appeared similar on the surface. This is why my story is based on an experience I had leading a psychoeducational group for the adult family members of persons with schizophrenia, all of whom were (like me) middle class and White. The challenges I faced in leading this 9-week group were related to differences that emerged in members' ages, gender, and religious beliefs. The implications of these differences for group cohesion became apparent at the beginning of the group (the normally calm preaffiliation phase) and persisted through the _power and control_ stage, before tapering off during the shared working and separation stages.

My family education and support group was a popular, recurring program offered at a community mental health center. Through lectures and discussion I attempted to provide the 6 to 12 members with education about schizophrenia and its related challenges to a fulfilling family life and help them develop social and resource supports, coping skills for dealing with their challenges, wider emotional support, and techniques for self-advocacy. Topics covered in the program included the range of services available for persons with schizophrenia; current theories about the causes, course, and treatment of the disorder; the uses and limitations of medications; and the various psychosocial interventions commonly provided in mental health agencies. I had learned over time that the primary therapeutic factors available in this group were the installation of hope from other members, member learning from interactions, the universalizing of each person's experiences, and acceptance by others.

One significant element of member diversity pertained to age. The members ranged in age from the mid-thirties through the seventies, and most were parents.

They represented clients who were in first-episode through the chronic stages of schizophrenia. I noticed immediately that members with younger children (late teens through the twenties) were more hopeful about the disorder remitting, and their family members resuming a normal life. The older members, however, many of whom had experienced decades of unfulfilled hopes and shattered dreams, were often resigned to the chronic nature of the disorder and their family members' modest potential for change. They had been disappointed by the limited progress of their children, and some were bitter about the "false promises" of mental health professionals regarding the effectiveness of their interventions.

Age: "Oh, don't get your hopes up about that."

As a result of this difference in age perspective, the older group members tended to actively discourage the younger members from holding out hopes for recovery. Although all the people who attended the group were well meaning, their life experiences colored their attitudes and they came off as rather dismissive and arrogant to the younger members. This process worked directly against the "installation of hope" therapeutic factor. As one example, Greta was pleased to announce one day that her 21-year-old son's psychotic symptoms had largely remitted, and he was planning to re-enroll in college soon. Another member responded, "Oh, don't get your hopes up about that. He'll never be the same. It's best that you accept the fact now."

One of my roles in the group, in response to interactions like this, was to remind the members that each client is different; that there is no predicting a final outcome with schizophrenia, though it was likely that some symptoms of the disorder would persist. I was always upbeat in my presentations but could not help but notice that the younger members sometimes felt "stung" by the rebukes of the older members, and lost some of their enthusiasm for the group. Although the older members' tendencies to temper the hopes of younger members may have provided appropriate learning to some degree, it was also demoralizing at times in a way that ran contrary to the goals of the group. Still, the "learning from interactions" factor was sometimes enhanced in these exchanges, as the older members were able to share the coping skills they had developed over the years and particularly encouraged the younger members to be assertive in their interactions with professionals.

Gender: "You'll never know what it's like..."

Another element of diversity in the group is that men and women participated, though there was always a majority of women, and they seemed to share the experience of most responsibility falling onto their shoulders for keeping their family systems as conflict free as possible. They tended to harbor some resentment toward the male members and to see their efforts to support the client family member as half-hearted. "You'll never know what it's like to live or die with the status of your child like I do," was one member's "reassuring" comment to a male member. "I had to be a full-time caregiver while my husband stayed at work or went out with his friends," she said, implying that the male member was somehow like her husband. These comments worked against my desired "acceptance by others" theme. My interventions at this time involved praising all those who had chosen to come to the group and pointing out the ways in which they had all shown love for their child relatives. As a male I was sensitive to the positions of the men and promoted their status as caring family members. At the same time, I noticed that some men were somewhat reluctant to speak out as a result of the female-dominated culture of the group.

Religious belief: "You need to engage in a lot more prayer..."

Thirdly, religious belief was diverse in the group, in that approximately one half of those who attended were highly religious, and found great comfort in their beliefs, whereas the other one half was less so. Those who maintained strong religious affiliations, especially the older members, had come to rely on their faith to get them through hard times with their client family members. They tended to offer suggestions to all members' concerns about everyday challenges, ongoing family conflicts, and the stress of having a person with mental illness in the family, with religious themes, such as, "You need to engage in a lot more prayer at a time like this," "Look to your pastor for comfort," or "Do you encourage your daughter to go to church?" Although these suggestions were generally accepted positively, the concerned member may have been looking for concrete, practical advice about, for example, motivating a child to attend vocational rehabilitation services, and they tended to tune out the religion-based comments of some others. Again, my role was to emphasize the many possible coping strategies that family members could constructively develop to enhance the quality of their lives, and that not all strategies worked well for everyone. Toward this end I framed religious comments as being one reflection of the universal search for meaning and purpose in light of major stressors.

The impact of these three types of diversity did not necessarily produce active conflicts among the members. I rarely perceived that an occasional negative interaction resulted in a member dropping out of the group (though it probably did so at times), but these three interacting differences did set group processes in place that made some members initially wary of others. Still they did not prohibit a shared working stage from developing. It was helpful for me to keep Yalom and Leszcz's (2005) therapeutic factors in mind and relate all member contributions to these broader themes. The group course was offered three times per year at my agency, and I never felt that it might be necessary (or would be possible) to reconfigure the criteria for group admission based on any demographic characteristics. Rather, I needed to be prepared for these common themes and address them in my own presentations to members, including my pregroup phone interviews that served as an orientation to new members and addressed the range of experiences sources of support that would be evident among the members. When I reviewed the group evaluations at the end of each course I was reminded that the goals of the program were being achieved, and I was reminded that one of my functions as the leader was to identify all types of diversity present (as much as I could, because of course some diversities are invisible) and help all members come together.

References

Yalom, I. D., & Leszcz, M.. (2005). *The theory and practice of group psychotherapy* (5th ed.). New York, NY: Basic Books.

Celebrating Neurodiversity: An Often-Overlooked Difference in Group Work

Barbara Muskat

For many years I worked in a children's mental health center, supporting children and youth with learning disabilities, and their families. To qualify for services, the children and youth had to be officially diagnosed with a learning disability, attention-deficit/hyperactivity disorder, or autism spectrum disorder (ASD) in addition to struggling with psychosocial issues. These diagnoses offered confirmation to families that something was "wrong" with these children. The majority of families brought their children to the center to address what were seen as "deficits," to improve social skills, or to address behavioral problems, essentially to "fix" their children. Therefore, as a member of the agency's staff, I was part of those who thought we should be "fixing" these kids and helping them socialize, communicate, and ultimately behave "like everyone else," despite the strengths-based approach of the programs offered by the center (weekly groups, summer camps, and individual and family counseling).

During the 20 years that I worked at the agency, quite a bit changed in the field of disability. Although disabilities were once seen through the lens of the medical model, as flaws or imperfections that required fixing; nowadays the lens of the social model is prevalent, which views disability as part of the diversity of the human condition. This has expanded to include the neurodiverse, who identify as having neurological, cognitive or behavioral differences, in particular ASD.

Applying the social model of disability to the children I worked with at the agency did not happen when I worked there, however it has led me to rethink a group experience that took place almost 20 years ago in the children's mental health center that I described above. The group was offered for boys with learning disabilities, psychosocial struggles, and features of ASD. At the time, there was far less known about ASD, diagnosis was imprecise and included a number of different labels. Children with features of ASD were often poorly understood, socially excluded, and unable to find peers who would understand and accept them.

The 9-week group comprised six boys, ages 10 to 13, and two female facilitators. I was the supervisor of the group, observing from behind a one-way mirror. I also knew most of the boys from my work with them and their families.

"Are you a TTC-er?"

My experience with the boys was that they wanted to interact with others, share experiences, and have fun, but in their lives outside of the group their individual quirky ways of interacting would get in the way. For example, an intense interest in the city's transportation system was common to the boys, which they loved to discuss with anyone who would listen. When the group began and they introduced themselves to each other, one of the more vocal boys asked in a demanding voice of each of the other members, "Are you a TTC-er?" meaning: were they obsessed with the Toronto Transit Commission. It was imperative to the inquiring boy that they all share this important aspect of his life, and he urgently needed to know this about each of the other group members. In this case it turned out that indeed, they were all TTC-ers!

As well they could become very silly, ask lots of questions to others, would not understand if they were invading the personal space of others, or would fully withdraw if the noise level became too loud. This was all tolerated by the boys when in the group, whereas in the rest of their lives this led to being socially excluded, being bullied, and rarely having a say in how they were treated.

Group facilitation was guided by the belief in the importance of feeling accepted and understood by others, as well as by mutual aid. The boys' parents hoped that the group would help the boys to have a successful social experience as well as develop skills that would support them with social experiences outside of the group.

Each session started with a check-in about the boys' daily experience and ended with a wrap-up, to reflect on and summarize what happened in the group. Group leaders would have a theme prepared for each session, however they would also support the boys to raise issues and facilitate interaction. Activities were also planned to provide opportunities for the boys to have fun together with peers. The leaders would encourage the boys to participate in discussions and then to think about how they interacted with one another. And even though the group was not set up to "fix" the members, attempts were made to shape the members' behavior and to reflect on their member-to-member interaction.

The boys bonded quickly and recognized similar experiences, traits, and interests among themselves. They expressed a desire to be with others with similar interests and who wouldn't exclude or tease them. The boys would sometimes appear to not engage with one another, as they did not typically look at each other, would seem to not be listening, or would wander in the group room. However they would subsequently display indications that they were listening and responding to the other group members. The group members displayed acceptance of one another's distinct behaviors, like sitting too close or laughing too loudly or talking a lot about specific topics. They also offered each other understanding and support when discussing distressing peer interactions at school or in the community. When they were happy they would laugh and roll around, and it was very clear that they were happy. And when they spoke about something that upset them, they would be quieter and more solemn and clearly were upset.

The "F" word: "Feelings, feelings, feelings!"

In many interactions between the leaders and the members, the leaders, who were newly trained social workers, would duly ask the boys how they felt about what went on in the group at that time. Asking children how they felt about issues was a common approach at the time, with a hope that expressing feelings would offer some release of emotions that might otherwise have been held in. As children and youth with ASD are often described as struggling with identifying their feelings and those of others, this seemed particularly salient at the time. These boys had been asked how they felt about matters many times in their lives, and this was often experienced as challenging and frustrating to them.

In one session a boy discussed how difficult it was and how exasperated it made him when people asked him about feelings. This led to much talking and laughing among the boys about their similar experiences, culminating in their repeatedly saying the word *feelings*. The boys began chanting "feelings, feelings, feelings." They told one another that they did not want anyone to say that word in the group. They then called the word the "F" word. Subsequently when anyone would use a derivation of the word *feelings* the boys would yell together, "You said the word … you said the word." They would laugh together at these times, produce a unified response, and seemed to greatly enjoy having some control of this one aspect of their life in the group.

These expressions happened much to the consternation of the group leaders, who would have likely preferred that the boys express their "feelings" through calm discussion. The leaders would try to placate or settle the boys. As the group supervisor, I had some mixed feelings. I also wanted the boys to reflect on their experiences and express their thoughts, but I also was able to see the joint fun the boys were having in the moment. Furthermore, I was acutely aware of the presence of their parents in the waiting room, who were hoping that the group would help the boys interact more "normally." I did not want to be known as the group supervisor who did not control the behavior of her group members!

In hindsight, asking these boys to describe, discuss, and process a concept that was inherently challenging for them was likely experienced as belittling, even disrespectful to them. It perhaps added to the notion that they were somehow flawed and required fixing. However, in their coming together as a group they were empowered to speak their minds, advocate for themselves, and challenge the leaders to stop focusing on a concept that they were asked about too often in their lives. In essence, they were clearly communicating their feelings. The group offered the boys a chance to feel accepted and understood. Moreover, I believe it inadvertently provided them with an opportunity to assert an even greater degree of agency that in today's time might be praised as an affirmation of their neurodiversity. I now regret that the leaders and I did not celebrate this affirmation together with them.

"Cure neurotypicals now: Offended? Now you know how we feel"

When I think back about this group I often wonder if it were conducted today whether the purpose would still be to fix or enhance the boys' social behavior or whether the purpose would focus on supporting the boys to become ASD self-advocates, who accept their strengths and challenges, and develop enhanced self-perceptions as members of a neurological minority.

Adults with ASD are starting to challenge the negative stereotypes associated with autism. There is a now a website devoted to neurotypical syndrome (http://isnt.autistics.org), which is described as a common condition affecting individuals who are nonautistic. There have even been public relations campaigns with slogans like "Cure Neurotypicals Now: Offended? Now you know how we feel." From my perspective, I do not believe that this degree of neurodiversity has yet made its way to children and youth with ASD, as many parents are still desperately searching for a cure. This is evidenced by the mission statement of Autism Speaks, an organization devoted to improving the lives of individuals with autism, "We are dedicated to funding global biomedical research into the causes, prevention, treatments and a possible cure for autism."

Reflecting on this group experience has challenged me to consider my own biases about the work I do and to be mindful about how group purpose and individual and group goals are determined. Helping others to change should only take place if they believe change will benefit them, not just because they have been determined to fit a diagnostic category that is located outside of the typical world. Asking children and youth to work on changing traits that are hard wired into their being is a pretty colossal request!

I will end this reflection with the words found on a poster during Autism Awareness Week in 2005, likely developed by individuals with ASD and their family members. It fully reinforces a strength-based description, rather than dwelling in deficit. The poster reads "Autism Pride Day: There is no cure for being yourself." We all need to remember this when working with group members who are being themselves.

Come As You Are!: Creating Community with Groups

Melissa Eaton

A jackhammer pounds away at the concrete outside the front door of the drop-in center as I navigate between the orange construction cones, hopping over wet concrete to unlock the front door. It's a foggy Friday morning on 6th Street in San Francisco. 6th Street is a four-block overcrowded extension of the notorious Tenderloin neighborhood that disproportionately hosts the city's most marginalized and vulnerable residents. Many of them are currently homeless or at risk of homelessness and are dealing with mental health disorders and substance misuse. The single-room occupancy (SRO) hotels, the most ubiquitous housing option for people with low income, offer rooms with enough space for a bed and a sink with shared bathrooms in the hallway and are cramped against each other lining 6th Street. These SRO hotels have started charging $300 a week to stay in roach-, mouse-, and bed bug–infested rooms making even this option increasingly impossible. The tech boom that is gentrifying the city's most affordable neighborhoods is in full force on 6th Street, the jackhammer a constant reminder that the sudden "beautification" of this street will result in the squeezing out of the people who have called this historically inhospitable street home for decades.

The drop-in center where I work as a psychotherapist serves roughly 100 people a day who are currently experiencing homelessness and/or extreme poverty and are living on or near 6th Street. Services the drop-in center offers range from offering a cup of coffee, providing a comfortable chair in which to take a quiet nap, providing respite from the weather or police harassment, case management, employment search assistance, community-building activities like Bingo and movie days with popcorn, massage therapy, drop-in harm reduction psychotherapy and harm reduction drop-in group therapy. I work for the Center for Harm Reduction Therapy and am contracted to be at the drop-in center 4 days a week to provide individual and group therapy.

Harm reduction psychotherapy is a combination of psychotherapy and substance use treatment that allows clients to address their substance use and their underlying issues at the same time. It is a client–therapist collaboration that empowers clients to define and prioritize the goals they would like to work on, making reducing any current harmful behaviors the first order of business. Drop-in therapy is extremely low barrier because clients do not need an appointment, they can sign up that day to see someone.

Preparing

Our drop-in group therapy works with the same low barrier threshold as our individual therapy that means clients can attend group anywhere from 5 minutes to the entire hour, and no one is ever "late" to group. Our groups are flexible, and to call them diverse would be an understatement. Our group members consist of people who are active substance users, people who have been abstinent for 20 years and are staunch Alcoholics Anonymous (AA) members, people who come high on speed, come in to take an opiate-induced nap, come in to give themselves an extra hour in the morning before they start drinking beer, people whose extreme social anxiety or depression causes them much isolation in many other parts of their lives, people who are actively hearing voices and tell the group about what they hear when they hear it, senior citizens, transitional-age youth, Black, Latino, Asian Americans, White, gay, straight, bisexual, male- and female-identified people. We like to repeat the mantra, "Come as you are!"

Today is one of the 3 days a week we offer our Harm Reduction Drop-In Group. I have arrived early to plug in the coffee and organize the group room in the most soothing and comfortable way possible. I position the chairs so each person can have as much physical space as possible in our tiny room, adjust the lamp lights and turn off the fluorescents, put the fan on low, and spritz the air with some lavender water. I sit down, center myself, close my eyes, and take a few deep breaths inhaling deeply. Often group members come to group in different states of crisis, and I have learned quickly that my state of mind and calmness is crucial to the well-being of my group.

Checking in

As I open the door 10 minutes before group starts so people can settle in with coffee, all eight chairs are quickly filled. By the end of group today, 16 people will have attended. Miles, who is an active speed user, suffers from major depressive disorder, was just evicted from his housing, and usually can't stay seated longer than 10 minutes, grabs a cup of coffee and announces he is going to wait outside where there is more air until there is an open chair.

Shannon, a woman who has an extensive trauma history, a chaotic relationship with crack, and is an occasional group member, is having a difficult time fitting on the small round coffee table that becomes the ninth chair often in our group. Mark, a man with schizoaffective disorder who has been experiencing homelessness for decades and barely utters more than a few words in group, deftly picks up the lamp that is also on the table and sets in on the floor next to him so Shannon has more room to sit down.

Me:	Good morning group! Welcome everybody to Harm Reduction Drop-In Group. Just a reminder this is a drop-in group so people can come in and out as they like. I will help remind folks to share the talking time and please remember to ask permission before you give someone feedback. What did I miss, group?
Lance:	You can come high or you can come low!
Me:	That's right! Come as you are!
Christopher:	One person talks at a time.
Shannon:	If you get a cup of coffee you have to stay for the whole time.
Me:	Thanks, group! Great reminders. Shannon, I'm curious about that coffee rule.
Shannon:	(laughs a little). I know, it's not really a rule, but I think it should be. I think if you drink our coffee you should at least stay for as long as it takes you to drink it.
Christopher:	I think it's okay for people to get coffee and leave. That's how I started coming to this group.
Shannon:	Yeah, but maybe they would get even more out of it if they stayed longer!
Me:	Well, feel free to invite anyone who gets coffee to stay for the group. Are you okay with continuing to be our group's ambassador, Shannon?
Shannon:	(smiling) Yeah, I guess.
Me:	Okay, group! Who wants to check in today?
Jordan:	I do!
Lance:	I do!
Jordan:	(to Lance) You can go ahead, man.

Jordan is an anxious young man with bipolar disorder who comes to every group. He used to insist on checking in first, if he wasn't the first person to check in, he would go outside and smoke a cigarette until it was his time to check in, then he would leave group abruptly after he checked in, stating, "I don't want any feedback." After several months, he began letting certain group members he started to trust give him feedback. Once he saw what kind of feedback they offered him and felt supported, he started allowing feedback from the entire group. Presently in group he offers others the chance to check in before him, he stays in the room and listens to their check-ins, and he asks the group to give him feedback on his check-in when he is done.

Jordan used to be on probation when I first met him and had lost his housing for engaging in physical fights. He is now off of probation, has had no trouble in the past year and a half, and has maintained his housing. He often prides himself on the skills he has learned to deescalate and calm himself in the moment to avoid violent conflict. Because our groups have no expectations of how little or long people attend, it allows individuals like Jordan to build tolerance and attend group on their own terms. If Jordan had been expected to come to group every week and stay for the entire hour his anxiety would have prohibited him to come to group at all. There is rarely a group where he is not present.

Lance: I'm doing good today. I'm going to go play Bingo at the senior center with my friend later. They are serving pizza and soda and cake I think. They finally fixed my sink that was leaking so I got some sleep last night. Oh yeah and the Giants are playing tonight! So I'll watch the game with some of my neighbors in the community room.

Shannon: Who are they playing?

Lance: The Dodgers.

Jordan: Go Giants! Okay it's my turn to check in. I'm doing really good today. I'm thinking about a lot of things. I'm trying to stay positive and trying to let go of other people's ideas of who I am. I'm trying not to worry about the negative thoughts and comments some people have about me (goes into more detail for another minute).... If anyone would like to give me feedback I'm open to it.

Miles: (who just came in and found a seat at the beginning of Jordan's check-in) You're always gonna have haters and celebrators. Listen to the celebrators and screw the haters. (gets up and exits group again)

Lance: Keep up the good work, Jordan. You are smart and talented and you have a lot going for you. Don't listen to those negative people.

Timothy: Oh, me, me! I want to check in. Today I'm thinking about the presidents of the United States of America. You have Hoover who was a real dingbat. John F. Kennedy was assassinated because of his liberal politics. Lincoln who used Black people as puppets to gain popularity. Which brings me to Obama...

My stomach is tightening as I wonder if I will need to interrupt him soon as he has made racist comments in the past and has worked very hard in group over the years to become much more accepting. I breathe a quiet exhale of relief as he finishes his check-in uninterrupted and without offending anyone.

Timothy has fixed delusions about the government and social services, and though he has permanent housing, he sleeps outside most nights because of his paranoia. I usually offer him feedback first as the group has a difficult time relating to him. I will make a comment like, "Wow, it's really amazing how much you can remember! You are like a walking encyclopedia!"

Freddie: (breaks the silence. He turns his body toward Timothy giving him eye contact) You're a really smart guy and I really enjoy your check-ins.

Timothy: (sits quietly and smiles big)

Freddie, a man with schizoaffective disorder who lived for a decade under the freeway in a cardboard box and has a difficult time maintaining his (supplemental security income) benefits because he cannot remember to go to his appointments is sitting next to Timothy. I constantly have to remind Freddie to ask permission before giving feedback but did not want to intrude upon this sweet exchange.

Steve: Can I give you feedback?

Timothy: Yes.

Steve: I've been seeing you around for a while and I really like what you check in about and I think you're really intelligent.

I have never seen Timothy smile so big. My supportive feedback has certainly never touched him like this. For once he is at a loss for words and finally says, "Thanks, thanks!" through his broad smile. Timothy is very isolated in many parts of his life. His paranoia interferes with his ability to trust and form relationships with people and limits him to having few service providers he trusts. He has found support in this group that he does not have elsewhere.

Christopher: I'll check in next. I used last night and I'm feeling really bad about it. I'm also feeling pretty sick because of it too. Like a double whammy. I feel like a hypocrite because I've been going to church and getting counseling from the pastor there. I'm sorry if I'm short with people today. I just am in pain and feel really bad.

Me: Christopher, how do you feel about getting some support from the group?

Christopher: Yeah, I guess I would like some.

Jordan: Don't beat yourself up, man. It happens.

Shannon: Today is a new day, Christopher. It's okay.

Mark: I've known you for a long time and you are a man of God. You've helped me lots by listening to you.

Christopher: Thanks, man. That means a lot.

Freddie: I got these vitamins you can take! They will make you feel amazing! (starts pulling out some pills)

Me: Freddie, you are really trying to help Christopher out I can see. Remember this is a talking group, not a doing group.

Freddie: Oh, yeah, sorry. (puts the pills away)

Me: Christopher, slips are part of the process. We learn from them and then move on. It doesn't change who you are as a person.

It's clear your group members think a lot of you by the way they have supported you today.

Christopher: Thanks. Yeah, I know. Thanks guys.

Juan: (yelling out the group room door) Hey, It's Charles! (steps out of the room into the hallway to tell Charles that group is happening now).

Charles is a man with schizophrenia who rarely bathes and wears the same clothing most of the time, his paranoia prevents him from taking medication, and he has been dropping into group a few times a month for several years. Juan has obsessive compulsive disorder and has no relationships outside of the group, he comes to every group and stays the entire hour. He spends most of his time organizing his paperwork and making phone calls to the Social Security Administration to confirm his benefits.

Juan: (one foot in the group room, propping the door open) Hey, Charles, we are in group now! Come in to group!"

Charles: (enters group quietly, smiling, and gets coffee)

Juan: Charles, do you want to check in?

Charles: Yeah, okay. I've been calling my brother in Jersey, but he's not at home. I don't have any mail coming in. My son is on Jupiter, and he is not coming back to see me on my birthday. I ate some shark meat today, it filled me up pretty good, and I've been roasting coffee at home. I'm kind of easy going and heavy. I've been making the heat swell and swelter. Someone's going to listen to me. I just can't keep up with these coffee beans.

Me: Sounds like there is a lot going on, are you feeling some stress?

Charles: (smiles) No, I'm feeling breezy.

Me: Well, I'm really glad Juan reminded you about group and you decided to come in. It's always good to see you here.

Juan: Good to see you, Charles.

Freddie: Here, Charles, I brought you these. (hands him a fleece jacket in good condition and a pair of pants)

Charles: (smiling) Thank you.

Me: Wow, Freddie, how thoughtful of you. Mark, would you like to check in today?

Mark is the man with schizoaffective disorder who moved the lamp off the table to accommodate Shannon in the beginning of group. Mark comes to almost every group. He nods his head in understanding and mumbles to himself throughout the group but rarely speaks or checks in. When he decides not to check in I thank him for modeling to the group that it is okay not to check in and it's important to have listeners in the group.

Mark: Not really, I don't have much to say. I come to this group to be around people. That's it.

Christopher: Yeah, me too. That's why I come too.

Me: I bet you two are not the only ones who come to group for that reason. You are very supportive of others in this group, Mark. You give a lot of nonverbal feedback by listening closely and nodding your head a lot.

Mark: Yeah, I really like what other people say in here. I like listening to them and thinking about how it is for me too.

We are halfway through the group and almost everyone has checked in. Steve, a man with major depression who recently lost his father and is a sporadic crack user has been quiet most of the group which is unusual for him.

Steve: I want to check in. I am really pissed off. Somebody stole my father's watch from my room. I think I know who it is and I'm trying really hard not to go kick his ass. But it's taking everything I have not to go find him and beat him up. (he starts to cry which he has never done in group before)

Shannon: Do you want some feedback?

Steve: (through tears) Yeah, okay.

Shannon: That is terrible that someone you thought was your friend stole from you. But, don't let him get you in trouble. You can't go beating him up because then you might go to jail.

Juan: I'm sorry your father's watch was stolen. That is really sad.

Freddie: Someone I thought was my friend stole my dog from me once. I never got over that. I still miss that dog. He went with me everywhere.

Timothy: Hey, Hey! I've got it! Why don't you get a mental patient from the psych ward to have sex with the guy and steal your father's watch back? Then the mental patient can kill him and claim insanity!

Steve: (bursts out laughing through tears) Thanks, guys.
The entire group is joining him in laugher.

Me: (speaking over the continued laughter) Group, everyone is laughing at Timothy's hilarious and very insensitive joke but that's not really the plan is it?

Shannon: Oh come on, Melissa! You know he was joking!

Me: okay, okay, just checking. You know, I've got my license and all on the line here.

Timothy laughs along with the group and smiles big again. He gave Steve what he really needed in that moment just like Steve had encouraged him after his check in at the beginning of group.

Creating a culture of kindness

I started leading these groups with the belief that creating a culture of kindness, acceptance, and strength-based feedback would cultivate unique and supportive relationships. Now I have evidence that it works. As the group leader, I model commenting on the strengths in every group member, but when the supportive statement actually comes from another group member, it has a more powerful effect. The smiles are bigger, the pride is deeper, and the connection is more solid when another group member offers the words that someone else in the group really needs to hear.

As I sat in my office reflecting on this foggy Friday morning group, I came to tears. I spend my days commuting on buses and trains with people whose eyes never leave their phones. It is so refreshing to witness my group members offer genuine care and support to one another. I have seen them share their last box of cereal because they cannot bear the thought of their fellow group member feeling hungry as they have been before. I don't want to glorify poverty in any way. I witness the inhumane suffering that many of my clients endure and have endured for decades. It has been life changing for me personally and professionally leading the Harm Reduction Drop-In Groups. My group's care for each other gives me hope in humanity.

LANGUAGE

"The greatest obstacle to international
understanding is the barrier of language."
Christopher Dawson

"Professors, Why Did You Ask Us to Throw Out All Our Hopes and Dreams?"

Carol S. Cohen and Yuxin Pei

Introduction

Working with multiple languages in group work is a challenge, bringing a host of considerations for members and workers. Although a simple error in translation is at the heart of the episode presented here, we believe this story goes far beyond language fluency and tells how a single phrase would lead to confusion, despair, compliance, courage, and ultimately cross-cultural understanding and expanded competence. This event took place in 2012 as part of a workshop sponsored by the Department of Social Work and Sociology of Sun Yat-Sen University in Guangzhou, China.

This article continues with the story of what happened. We were fortunate that much of the session was videotaped and we referred to this in writing this report. Following the vignette, our article then discusses what we and the students learned from this experience and how it continues to influence our ongoing partnership. Our purpose is to illuminate some of the common and different aspects of social work with groups and professional education around the world through cross-cultural group work collaboration.

The workshop

With a focus on social work with groups, the proposed topics for the full-day workshop were curriculum development, supervision, and emerging trends in social work regulation. Upon arrival, we discovered a couple of things that called for a change in plans. Instead of the experienced practitioners and educators we were expecting, participants were current students and recent graduates, including a few of Yuxin's current students. As Yuxin recalls, "I felt sorry for not having enough experienced social workers in attendance, and feeling hopeful that the group could work well even though we had more students." Although finding this a bit disconcerting, Carol shared that she felt they could work through this together. We quickly conferred and agreed on needed changes. As soon as we began, we noticed that most of the participants were not sufficiently fluent in spoken English to conduct the workshop without translation of Chinese/English. Yuxin was then unexpectedly put in the position of translator.

We began the workshops with introductions and asked participants to share what interested them most about group work. Based on their contributions, we contracted with the group to focus on potential benefits of groups, components in understanding group work and planning groups, and working through challenges in the group as well as in the organizational or community context. Our morning session included activities designed to engage participants and encourage sharing of their experiences, concern, or questions. Each activity was processed, using the workshop group as an example of a task group convened to learn more about group work. Activities and discussion were "low demand" in that content of members' contributions were voluntary (though everyone was encouraged to participate), activities were fully explained before they started, and questions focused largely on professional development, rather than personal experiences.

We advised the workshop participants that we would "do" and "talk" about group work as the day unfolded, based on their experience and interest. The participants appeared to enthusiastically participate in the morning session, and we broke for lunch with good feelings. We had overcome quite a bit—the completely different composition of the participants, the unanticipated requirement for full translation, and the need to rework a day's agenda in the moment.

The throw it out activity

Carol's narrative

Based on how engaged the workshop participants became during activities in the morning, I proposed reconvening after lunch with an exercise that seemed appropriate to the midpoint, requiring a bit more individual investment. After welcomes and contracting for the afternoon session, we began the activity by asking participants to think about something that is "holding them back from being "great group workers," and asked each of them to think of one thing they are willing to share with the group that "they would like to get rid of." I suggested that they could metaphorically experience what it would be like to "throw out" what was holding them back through this activity. When using this type of activity in past, group participants seemed to relish such a prospect. I cannot say that these participants were excited by this idea, but they appeared to thoughtfully consider what they would "throw out."

Next, I asked participants to pantomime throwing something into the center of the room and say what the item was that "seemed to be holding them back." The participants began a bit hesitantly, although all contributed. Among the items thrown into the center were "solidarity, happiness to help people, self-development, and social change." I recall being somewhat confused by their choices. In one instance, I tentatively interpreted one participant's choice of "wanting to be a great group worker," as perhaps being held back by high expectations; another passing thought was that participants might feel uncomfortable about sharing what they saw as a deficit. Yuxin and I acknowledged their contributions. Some quizzical looks were made by participants during the throwing part. When completed, I invited the participants to join in "gathering all the refuse into bundles." With my encouragement, we pretended *to "sweep up" and then "fill and tie the bags."* We all went to the exit with the bundles and dramatically threw them out the door, and slammed it shut. Possibly caught up ourselves in the moment and wanting the activity to go well, Yuxin and I participated with a sense of play.

We then returned to our room. Instead of expected laughter and smiles, the participants were rather reserved. I asked what they thought of the activity. At first a couple of participants said they enjoyed the pantomime aspects. When the group became silent, I observed, "You are all pretty quiet about this," and then asked, "Why do you think that is happening?" As in our title, one bold participant asked, "Professors, why did you ask us to throw out our hopes and dreams?" I thought, "Oh my—What next?" Quickly sharing that I had thought they would "throw out their obstacles," I immediately heard Yuxin explaining that she misunderstood, and thus made an error when translating. The humor of the situation was inescapable, yet I felt I was witnessing something very special with Yuxin's admission, a turning point that might lead to a much deeper discussion than I had anticipated.

Yuxin's narrative

At the beginning of the exercise, I asked the participants to think what was "holding them in being a great social worker?" or in other words, "What was contributing to them being a great social worker?" I felt it was a very good question. And then when Carol asked everyone to throw these things into the center of the room, I still didn't feel there was anything wrong. According to my understanding, I thought Carol wanted the participants to know that what made you feel good about being a great social worker probably also hindered you to be a great social worker, and that's why you had to throw them, and restart yourself. So I translated Carol's instructions, without any questioning, because I interpreted Carol's instructions according to my understanding. When Carol asked the participants to pretend to take a broom and dustpan to collect the "rubbish they had thrown out, and then take the bundles outside," I just felt that she was very humoros because I didn't think she would say this to be humiliating. I felt surprised that the participants seemed reluctant to "throw out" what they had, and I thought they were probably too young to understand the oriental philosophy of "broken off," meaning that you should reconsider what you have and treasured, as you may not need them as you think—abandoning them sometimes can make you even more effective and happier.

I recognized the problem when we began the sharing session, when a participant asked, "Professors, why did you ask us to throw out all our hopes and dreams?" and Carol said that she never asked them to do that, and instead asked them to throw out what "held them back from being a great social worker." I realized that I misunderstood the sentence and gave wrong instructions to the participants, which made the workshop proceed into an opposite direction as Carol proposed. I felt very awkward because I would "lose face" in front of my students, ex-students, and colleagues. But I knew I had to tell everyone what a mistake I had made, otherwise everyone would feel confused about what happened in the group, and the true ideas of Carol's design had to be explained. When I then spoke out about the mistake, I felt relieved. Everyone laughed, but I didn't think they were laughing at me. I felt okay about making mistakes and admitted them, as long as I still could do something to repair the mistakes.

Retrieving all our hopes and dreams

As we began to rewind what had happened, the participants expressed feeling released from their concern and confusion. We thanked the student who asked the critical question, which was echoed by participants. Carol said that she greatly appreciated Yuxin's effort in doing this workshop together and admired her humility and strength in explaining what had happened. The participants showed their respect to Yuxin for speaking out the mistake in such a situation. They said they appreciated it very much, as not every professor would be likely to do that in front of their students.

The participants shared that even when they were in a pantomime, they were really into their own roles. They felt so confused and reluctant to throw out "what they treasured," which made them upset and not cheerful at all. They couldn't understand why Carol used such a joyful voice, facial expression, and body language to encourage them to do what they didn't want to do. But, they reported, they just did what they were asked to do. On the other hand, they reported that If Carol had not "insisted" that they give feedback on what happened in the whole group after they had built a kind of connection and trust with Carol in the morning, they would probably have not confided their thoughts and worries at all, and the process of the group would have gone in another direction.

Following this discussion, Carol asked the group if they were willing to "play some more." All agreed, and everyone was invited to stand up and go to the door. We went outside, and at Carol's urging, "searched for the bundles we had thrown out." When we found them, participants "hoisted them on their backs" and brought them into our room. Great drama accompanied the "untying of the bundles" and the glow of the "precious hopes and dreams." We considered whether to randomly distribute the items in the bundles, and the group decided they should be returned to their original owners for review. Participants were able to treasure, as well as reflect on their meaning. This final element set the stage for the fuller and illumining discussion of the interplay of expectations, barriers, and skills in becoming effective group workers from the member and worker perspective. As we planned together at the beginning of the workshop, our agreement to "do" group work and "talk" group work served us well. The shared experiences brought a higher level of engagement, and we were able to discuss cultural differences and similarities in practice approaches, what each of us learned from the day, and our plans to work towards putting our learning into action.

Discussion and summary

Confusion

As highlighted in our story, confusion about the activity and instructions was evident even as it was introduced. Yuxin and Carol thought of this as normal because the students were being drawn into an unfamiliar type of learning. We each found ways to understand what we were observing and, as it turned out, made premature interpretations. We could have clarified and asked participants how they understood the tasks. We were open to answering questions but did not explicitly invite them. It is only in retrospect that we have considered the impact of the extraordinary complicating (and perhaps confusing) factors for the participants in the workshop, given the last minute changes we had to make in the program and unexpected need for full translation.

Despair

Clearly, we did not fully identify the shift of many participants from confusion to despair and discomfort. To some extent we were occupied by explaining and lost some ability for tuning into the moment. For Carol, this was complicated by a diminished facility to read behaviors and affect in this novel Chinese context, and a concern about offense if an embarrassing behavior was exposed. For Yuxin, commitment to the task of translation and desire to help Carol "save face," caused her to go forward through some misgivings. The participants certainly were in a less powerful position than we were. As they shared in the debriefing process, many felt caught in a "no-win" situation in which they experienced sadness while throwing away their hopes yet felt either that they did not have the power to protest, or that some reason for the instructions would eventually be revealed. Upon reflection, we feel that there are broad differences between China and the United States in this regard. However, the lesson to keenly observe and stay with any group throughout its process was reinforced through this experience.

Compliance

We were delighted (and relieved) that the participants accepted our suggestions for the workshop agenda in the morning and thought we had done a fairly good job of contracting given our limited time to plan the purpose and content for the day. The students and early professionals in the workshop were happy to attend the session, and had heard about Dr. Cohen, the Fulbright Scholar from the United States, leading the workshop. Many knew and admired Dr. Pei from classes and the Department of Social Work and Sociology. As Yuxin recalled, "They didn't think these professors would make mistakes." When combined with the participants' very limited experience of being expected to share even filtered feedback, we collectively contributed to a "perfect storm" of compliance.

Courage

Our "hero" in this story is the young man who exposed the problem. Once it was out, the participants were visibly relieved, and Yuxin's brave declaration substantially released the tension. Participants were exposed to two unusual events, as they were not used to questioning what professors were doing and were not expecting to hear professors admitting to mistakes and inviting discussion. Fortunately, they had seen glimpses of this in the morning, as Yuxin and Carol conferred, questioned, and engaged the members in analysis of the group process and their observations about leadership in our workshop group. We now see how this experience could be empowering and confusing for the participants. We did not use the incident to explicitly challenge prevailing relationships in the academy, though Yuxin's disclosure and community building approach, as well as Carol's trust and expectation of engagement served as models of other ways of working. Rather, we used the event to lead us to discussion of roles and interventions, and the theme of worker authority in social work practice. We engaged in considering how admitting mistakes and asking hard questions within a supportive context of mutuality might be considered signs of courage in social group work.

Cross-cultural understanding and expanded competence

For all of us, the Throw it Out incident and the discussions that followed brought a greater understanding of communication across distance. Perhaps fueled by Yuxin's sense of responsibility and humility, and Carol's sharing of her own confusion and worries, the participants were able to reflect on cross-cultural communication, particularly when intersectional issues of power are present. We looked at how cultural norms of members of groups with diverse composition and diversity between members and workers have a critical affect on group process. We also focused on assumptions made about culturally linked behaviors, especially when we share similar cultural (and other) characteristics with members. Our in vivo experience was a powerful touchstone in these discussions.

The episode was a valuable bridge into issues of power and worker control in the group, an area of discussion that can be difficult in settings with strong central authority structures. We were able to look at how these elements are ever present in practice, and that we must leave space open to see how they affect the group and its members. Our experience taught all of us that we must always cultivate the openness to be surprised, and resist automatic thoughts and explanations. Yuxin and Carol left the day with renewed appreciation of the workers' role in moving into new and sometimes difficult territory with members. At the same time, we became acutely mindful of how members are often heroes and catalysts.

In closing, the dramatic moments and ultimately positive outcomes contributed to the ongoing relationship Yuxin and Carol have developed. The unexpected need for translation may have brought us closer, as we were in some ways speaking for, and trying to understand each other on a deeper level than anticipated. We were tested by this experience, through which participants witnessed our reactions, our investment in the process, and ultimately our skills. Our final discussions of the workshop showed that the participants had taken it all in—the Chinese, the English, the spoken and the unspoken. For us, it was a profound experience of international collaboration and learning.

Acknowledgments

We thank the following organizations for their invaluable roles in making this workshop and collaboration happen:

The Department of Social Work and Sociology at Sun Yat-Sen University for supporting the collaboration and guest scholar visit, with special thanks for the facility and videotaping arrangements for the workshop; The Adelphi University School of Social Work and students for their encouragement and interest as this project unfolded; And, the 14 participants in the workshop at Sun Yat-Sen University, in appreciation for their enthusiasm, and openness, and thoughtful contribution.

Funding

The authors would like to thank the U. S. Fulbright Specialist Grant Program for supporting Carol S. Cohen's visit to China and the Hong Kong Polytechnic University's China Research and Development Network Centre for arranging and funding her visit to Guangzhou.

Working with a Diversity of Languages: Francophone and Anglophone Coparticipants in Groups of Parents of Transgender Children

Annie Pullen Sansfaçon and David Ward

It is well known that the parents of children who are transgender often struggle to find resources to meet their needs. When we obtained funding from the Social Sciences and Humanities Research Council of Canada to conduct research to better understand experience of parents of children who are transgender in Montreal, we were far from knowing that this project would lead to the development of a long-lasting group that still meets on a monthly basis today, where diversity of experience, and of language, have become hallmarks of the group

Both of us were working on the project. One had a role of consultant and the other, the role of lead researcher for the pilot project. The lead researcher on this project being a parent of an child who is affirmed transgender, we were closely attuned to the high level of discrimination and oppression experienced by those families. On that basis, we decided to develop the project using a methodology that would be empowering for its participants and, thus, to set up a community-based Participatory Action Research Project, that would draw on self-directed groupwork, an approach developed by Audrey Mullender and Dave Ward during the early 1990s, that is known to promote empowerment, at structural and personal levels for participants.

Getting started

During the planning phase of the group, we provided training to the research assistants who would cofacilitate the group. It was decided at this time that research assistants (RAs) would collect data to avoid any appearance of conflict of interest on the part of the researcher/parent of a child.

The training offered to RA was provided by using the self-directed groupwork principles and process so that participants could get a hands-on experience of the process, before facilitating the parents group. After having worked on the preplanning phase where the RAs/cofacilitators explored their value base and its coherence with self-directed groupwork principles, we moved on to the initial planning of the group. At that point of time, the objectives of the group were largely influenced by the research questions and focused on getting a deeper understanding of parenting a child who is gender creative or trans. During the third training session with the research assistants, we began to plan the first meeting with parents. In line with the principles of self-directed groupwork, we agreed that first meeting with potential group members should be as open as possible, providing only the minimum information so that potential group participants could decide whether they wanted to get involved. It was also agreed that the group would be held in the Montreal area, and that a community setting, as opposed to a university one, would offer a safer and more relaxed space for the first meeting.

Grappling with language diversity in the group

Montreal, being a city in the province of Quebec where French is considered the official language, but where a large Anglophone community lives, we agreed that it was essential to reflect on how we should envisage the language component in the group. Although we did not want to plan too much content, to let participants take core decisions during the first meetings, we wondered whether we should plan one group (bilingual) or two groups (unilingual) to start with. Indeed, according to self-directed groupwork principles, group work facilitators, in being committed to social justice, should ensure access to everyone who wished to participate; in the same vein, we strive to challenge oppression and, given the long struggle many Francophone citizens have experienced to maintain French as the official language,[1] the group would also need to promote a safe environment for Francophone as well as for the Anglophone participants. Indeed, Quebec has had a long history of oppression with regard to language and, for many years, Francophones have felt that they need to protect their language from North American English language domination. At the same time, some Anglophone communities in Montreal may also feel oppressed within this large Francophone community.

Hence, because of the specific cultural and historical context of Montreal city, some questions emerged with regard to language. A bilingual group could spark some issues of access, as some Francophones could feel uncomfortable participating where Anglophone are present, and vice and versa. Also, as little literature is available on how to facilitate bilingual groups, empirical evidence as to how best facilitate these types of groups is not widely available.

Nevertheless, undertaking two groups, that is one in French and one in English, was also far from straightforward. The resources were limited to two RAs who were able to work only a limited number of hours and the number of potential participants at the start of the project in 2011 was quite low. Indeed, at this time, the topic of children who were transgender was still considered very taboo and, therefore, we did not know many potential parents-participants would attend at the start of the project. Setting up two groups was therefore potentially problematic.

It was, therefore, during this planning meeting that the team had a long, sometimes heated, discussion. What was particular interesting, in hindsight, were the different ideas and arguments presented by each member during the discussion. The difference of opinion was stark between the Francophones (three of them, including a cofacilitator), versus the English speakers participants (two, including a cofacilitator) who took part in the training. After lengthy discussion, the team decided to advertise the group, circulate the invitation in both languages, and wait to see would turn up at the first meeting. Then, it was agreed, the cofacilitators would ask the participants what they thought about the language aspect of the group at the first meeting, and readjust according to the group decision. Although the most respectful way of embedding the self-directed groupwork principles into the planning of the intervention, this decision was not without its challenges, not least, that the cofacilitators would not know what to expect! However, they did have the reassurance of in depth consultancy planned to take place between group meetings.

Contracting: The group decides how to proceed

Contrary to expectations, at the first meeting, 14 parent-participants turned up. Most were bilingual, that is, they could communicate verbally in French or in English, with a minority of participants speaking only English. As planned, the cofacilitators discussed the language aspect of the group with the participants. Communication was offered largely in English at that point, but ideas spoken in French were translated by parent members to those who could not understand this language. At the end of the first meeting, the group had decided that the bilingual aspect was not a problem and that they would embed the question of the language directly into the group contract.

Central to the contract, the group decided that members should express themselves in their preferred language and that people who could not understand one or the other of the languages used would sit next to a bilingual member who would translate that part of the discussion that they did not understand. Upon reflection, this central feature of the group may have been central in fostering cohesion and in the development of mutual help among group members.

However, diversity about language did not stop at the first meeting, or in terms of the development of the social-affective life of the group. The bilingual nature of the group also fostered the development of a new vocabulary to talk about children and youth who are trans, which was very extremely limited in French at the beginning of the project. Indeed, during the first few meetings of the group, during the exploration of the question "What,"[2] group members started to stumble on defining who their children were; and, in describing them, they started by using a range of words and expressions to do so. Thus, the use of an appropriate term to describe their children's experiences also emerged as an important theme. The various expressions that can be used for this purpose and their meanings became a recurring topic across the sessions. Although there was no consensus about the use of one single term for the experience of their children, terms like "transgender," "gender creativity," "gender nonconformity," "gender independence," and "gender variance" were used widely among the group members. And what was particularly interesting is that those words were mainly in English. These discussions seemed important to parents as they occurred with regularity.

Finding the words together

Below is an excerpt of a discussion among parents about the use of terms to describe their children, recorded during the fifth meeting of the group (authentic scripts, with translation in brackets, when needed):

> [*Gender variance est un diagnostic. Et pour moi, je dirais que c'est la même chose [que non-conforme et créatif]*]. (Translation: Gender variance is a diagnosis. And for me, I would say that it is the same thing [as non-conforming and creative])
> [*Gender non-conforming, c'est négatif.*] (Translation: Gender nonconforming, it is negative)
> [*Créativité dans le genre, je ne me reconnais pas du tout. Mon enfant n'a pas d'intérêt pour les robes, pour le maquillage. Mais son corps, pour lui, c'est un cancer.*] (Translation: Talking about creativity related to gender, I don't recognize that myself, at all. My child has no interest in dresses, or for make up. But his body, for him, is like cancer)
> [*Créatif, je trouve ça mignon. Toutes les opportunités sont là.*] (Translation: Creativity, I think it is cute. All opportunities are available)
> [[*Gender variance*] *J'aime plus ça parce que c'est médical. Alors les gens ferment leur gueule. Bang! That's it, c'est médical.*] (Translation: Gender variance, I like it a lot because it is medical. So people shut their mouths. Bang! That's it, it is medical)
> [*Je n'aime pas gender variance. Il n'y a rien de médical là-dedans. Il est comme ça, c'est tout. Ce n'est pas une maladie. Creativity is good.*] (Translation: I don't like gender variance. There is nothing medical in this. He is like that, that is it. It is not a disease. Creativity is good)
> "That's the problem with the medical, you have to be a boy or a girl. There's no in-between."
> "I like more inclusive terms, so they don't have to fit in a box. Humans are complex. It's a complicated process to know somebody. It's not only about gender."

What is interesting to note, from this excerpt, is that not only does it illustrate the importance of bilinguism in the discussion, but also shows the frequent use of English terms to describe situations, even among Francophones. This highlights the sheer lack of vocabulary in French to express ideas related to naming the experience of parenting a child who is gender transgender. Indeed, at the start of this project, in 2011, there was a scarcity of research and information produced in French to discuss the lives and experience of children who were transgender. Because children who were transgender are in the midst of an identity development process and often do not identify themselves as "trans," finding the right terminology to discuss their children's experience was challenging for many.

As a result of this research and, particularly, the very rich discussions that took place in the parents group, the larger community of parents and people working with these families now have access to a vocabulary in French that has emerged from a bottom-up approach and reflects more truly the experience of families that support a child who is gender creative or trans.

Today, nearly 4 years after the end of the research group, the group continues to meet in Montreal, and the approach has begun to extend to other Canadian provinces.[3] It continues to be offered on a monthly basis, made of an open membership, with the language representation of participants roughly the same as at the beginning of the project (i.e., predominantly bilingual with some unilingual French and English participants).

Upon reflection, the bilingual aspect of the group has definitely contributed to the success and the continuity of the group. In addition to contributing to the development of a vocabulary, as the group went along, it has more than likely helped the development of the values of inclusiveness and social justice among group members. Continuing today, one of the core rules, when new members join, is that everyone is free to speak their preferred language, and that translation can be provided by comembers who sit around the table. As group workers and scholars who focus our work on group work, we would definitely promote the development of such groups.

Conclusion

Self-directed groupwork is a person-centered model rooted in antioppressive values and a vision of change that aims for social justice and emancipation. Self-directed groups have a distinctive collaborative commitment to achieving change on issues identified and owned by the group members themselves and that affects them all, across boundaries of diversity and intersectionality. Practitioners, as facilitators, are challenged to support the group and, without colonizing them, enable members to chip away at issues in their everyday lives—and, in the process, begin to question and deal with the forms of inequality that lie at the heart of current oppressive social arrangements.

The parents group has engaged with directly two such areas—children who are transgender and language diversity—both of which have gone largely unreported in the group work literature. The work and achievements of the group have demonstrated graphically the capacity of group work, if set in the goals of social justice, both to enhance the immediate lives of members and to promote new understandings and progressive social change in these areas.

Notes

1. See Noël, M. (n.d.) *Language Conflict in Quebec*. Retrieved from http://www.mccord-museum.qc.ca/scripts/explore.php?Lang=1&elementid=103__true&tableid=11&content long for brief history of French language conflict in Quebec.
2. Self-directed groupwork uses a question posing orientation in its intervention, which includes attention to the questions 'what is the chief concern," "why is it happening," and "how can it be changed / resolved."
3. For a full discussion about methodology and outcome of the research project, please see Pullen Sansfaçon, Ward, Dumais Michaud, Robichaud, and Clegg (2014).

Funding

This project was part of a bigger project funded by the Social Sciences and Humanity Research Council of Canada, Insight Development Grant, title "Princess Boys, Trans Girls, Queer Youth: Analyzing the Social, Educational, and Activist Worlds of Gender Nonconforming Children in Canada" obtained with Kimberly Manning, and Elizabeth J Meyer. Dave Ward acted as an adviser to the project. Annie Pullen Sansfaçon was the lead researcher for this specific component.

Reference

Pullen Sansfaçon, A., Ward, D., Dumais Michaud, A. A., Robichaud, M. J., & Clegg, A. (2014). Working with parents of gender variant children. Using social action as an emancipatory research framework. *Journal of Progressive Human Services*, *25*(3), 214–229.

Placing Diversity: Graduate Encounters with Group Work

Narine N. Kerelian

As a first generation Armenian-American growing up in California, I have been acutely aware of difference. I grew up with other dash-Americans. We had an unspoken sense of solidarity in the art of crafting our new identity pallets and being different together. I became acquainted with diversity through multicultural encounters that instilled in me a sense of wonder in being human in this world. The importance of the "placedness" of our experiences only became clear to me when I moved to Hong Kong. Despite my self-perceived openness to difference, I had unwittingly reified my North American "placed" multiculturalism and diversity, wanting to pack it in my suitcase and carry it across the Pacific.

The graduate encounter

The last time I can remember being assigned to be a member in a group in an educational context was when I was in middle school when I had the chance to select my own group members for class projects. That is, until I took my first graduate course in Hong Kong. As part of my graduate school core curriculum, I was required to take a course called Social Work and Applied Social Science Research Methods: Theory and Application. The professor assigned all the students to a research project on the topic of Mainland Chinese university students in Hong Kong and divided us into groups. We had to work together with each of our groups for the entire semester to produce a presentation.

The aim of this group was to put together a research puzzle by creating research questions, a brief literature review, a theoretical framework, selecting methodology, and implementing our proposal through a pilot study. We divided our group into parts of the project, where each group member took on a task (e.g., research questions, literature review, etc.). At the end of the course, each group was expected to combine all the parts into a group presentation.

I knew that this course was imperative to prepare us, PhD students, for our own research. The project was an invaluable exercise to enable us to learn the fundamentals of research. Nevertheless, I still had a tough time as I felt that I

117

lacked agency in the group member and topic selection process, as I did back in my middle school days. And the intercultural process was a challenge that I did not anticipate.

The umbrella movement and the right to vote

Being educated in the West, my desire was to choose who to work with in the group work and to have autonomy in selecting the topic for the research project. Furthermore, as I would learn, none of my cross-cultural trainings and lived experiences prepared me for this group. To frame the geo-political context of this experience, I was taking this graduate-level course as the Umbrella Movement was unfolding in Hong Kong with students taking to the streets to call for the democratization of Hong Kong's universal suffrage or right to vote.

At the end of September 2014, students organized a mass protest, known as the Umbrella Movement, by occupying roads outside of the government headquarters and in a few other key districts in Hong Kong to voice their concerns over what they thought of as a restriction on universal suffrage.

In 1997, Hong Kong transitioned from being a British colony to being a Special Administrative Region of The People's Republic of China. One of the stipulations in the handover to Mainland China was that universal suffrage was promised to the Hong Kong people. During the Umbrella Movement, major roadways were blocked for 79 days, the duration of the protest. Students camped in tents, gave talks, created make-shift areas for studying, and crafted political art to call for a more democratic Hong Kong.

As I walked through the protest grounds, I felt a sense of hope and despair all at once—hope because the students envisioned a better tomorrow and despair because of the powers in opposition to their movement. The true feelings of my graduate school Mainland group members were not clear to me. Even though we had a class discussion on the Umbrella Movement where some of my peers shared their thoughts, the restrictive political situation on the Mainland seemed to incite fear from being completely open about sentiments regarding their levels of participation in the protest in Hong Kong. I never really knew if they protested or not or even if they did attend the protests in secret because of the sensitivity of political activism in China.

A tense feeling lingered on campus. There were proponents of the movement who set up posters on the university's walls in support for democratizing Hong Kong, and opponents who took the posters down or posted counter statements. There was a deep need, yet seemingly few takers, to discuss the feelings of the different groups on campus: Mainland Chinese, Hong Kong Chinese, Hong Kong ethnic minorities, and international students. The dynamics of this turbulent political situation permeated the corridors of the university.

My fellow group members in the course included five students from Mainland China and one student from Hong Kong. From the start of our outside-of-class group meetings to divide the presentation sections of the group work, I picked up the role of the default group leader—in hindsight a role with cultural affinity—collecting each member's section, which included our interview tool, the literature review, methodology, research questions, and theoretical framework. No one objected to my volunteering as the group leader. As I started to receive the first few sections, I wrote an email to the group sharing my frank sentiments: "Everyone—I know we are getting a lot of comments from [professor], let's try to be as academically professional as possible when we do our sections. That means spelling/grammar/context, etc." (E-mail correspondence excerpt, November 2, 2014). This e-mail triggered a string of e-mails back and forth between me and the five Mainland Chinese students who had selected one student among them to represent their thoughts. The Mainland students thought that I had undermined their hard work by writing the e-mail noted above. The Hong Kong student read the e-mails as a neutral observer with one mediator type of reply, later sharing his feeling of being "caught" in the middle and questions regarding his identity in a post-handover Hong Kong. Even though Hong Kong is no longer a British colony, the identity of Hong Kong people is complex and appears ever shifting.

A change in leadership

In my understanding, some Hong Kongers feel a strong identity with a hybridized British Chinese orientation, some feel a Chinese identity linked to Mainland China, others a localized Chinese identity linked to Hong Kong, as well as identities in between and beyond the above-mentioned orientations. After numerous e-mails the Mainland students got together and decided to make Ming[1] the new group leader. I accepted their request as the course was coming to a close and all the sections had mostly been completed.

"Mandarin was spoken as if I did not exist in the room"

Although we all worked in a shared office, there was little verbal discussion until I approached the representative of the e-mails, Ming, and had a long conversation with her while sitting on the office floor near her cubicle. I reiterated that my intention was not for the Mainland colleagues to feel any personal offense from my e-mails, but that there seemed to be cultural differences being expressed by our different communication styles. I also confronted my unspoken grievances and feelings of isolation in our group meetings where Mandarin was spoken as though I did not exist in the room. It was not enough for me to think about my own cultural competency; I needed to communicate these thoughts with my colleagues to work through the challenges of our diverging expectations of what it meant to work together.

"My body acted quicker than my mind"

After having the long talk with Ming, I gave her a hug. My body acted quicker than my mind because my mind would have reminded me of the lack of "touch" as a tenet in interpersonal relations among Chinese colleagues, especially with foreigners in Hong Kong and the Mainland. However, I wanted to express the radical authenticity of my intentions with an affective gesture as an olive branch. Ming seemed to understand my gesture as she had previously studied in Canada and was aware of hugging in Western culture. Her reaction was to give me a few taps on my shoulder. I felt sincerity in her gesture, though it must have felt strange for her to be so direct. Ming seemed to also want to express reconciliation despite the awkwardness in the means of reciprocating it with some form of "touch."

How can what seems like a simple e-mail about checking our grammar become so convoluted in interpretation? The emotive dimensions of the political movement were penetrating our group's work without any explicit recognition of its impact on our work by the group, hindering the potential for cultivating authentic encounter. During the Umbrella Movement, there seemed to be a "you're either with us (Hong Kong people fighting for democracy) or against us (allied with the Chinese Communist Party and its constituents)" mentality.

Apart from Ming, the rest of the Mainland group members seemed to avoid contact with me even though we were in a shared office. They seemed comfortable with communicating their grievances with Ming who would then e-mail me their feelings and thoughts. However, when it came to face-to-face discussion about the issue, apart from a brief run-in with a female Mainland member of my group work, there was no meeting in person to discuss what had just happened until a few weeks later when the situation had cooled off. It takes bravery, trust, and a belief that there is something rewarding in opening up ourselves to other perspectives and realities.

Airing it out

Ming was brave enough to send me those e-mails to express her feelings and those of the Mainland students. She took the role as the messenger of the generally subjugated voices of Mainland students on campus who seem to be stuck between a rock and a hard place with the current political environment in Hong Kong, which appears bifurcated into proponents versus opponents of the Umbrella Movement. I wanted to articulate my point of view within my own value orientation just as much as my fellow group members wanted to express their own through the context of their cultural norms. By expressing difference, it felt like our roots were becoming unearthed and exposed by questions from those unfamiliar with each of our ways of knowing.

In retrospect, it was the pure state of vulnerability that became the wonder, the beauty of encounter, which made my group colleagues and I human together. The group took place in a territory with a transitional political system in the Asia-Pacific, which has aroused emotions from its denizens, as well as those in Mainland China. It is not enough to just "know" or be aware of different value orientations, but also to know something about the history of the places in which they take form and are practiced.

Learning in place

Reflecting on this critical incident awakened in me the importance of placedness in my understanding of diversity. The taken-for-granted assumptions about understandings and approaches for working in diverse groups do not clearly translate within all geo-social milieus. What this experience taught me was to treat every diversity experience as a new encounter, in its place. Being able to feel the richness of diversity also involves confronting its complexity with wonder, face-to-face with one another. Although diversity trainings are invaluable for broadening awareness, I was not prepared for the intricacies of this experience in Hong Kong. I learned only by living through them. I had perceived myself as a diversity proponent. In identifying in this way, I had become blind to the placedness of my diversity value orientations.

Engaging in diverse contexts does not mean giving up your unique sense of self, but it is about being able to translate your intentionality to cultivate a deeply trusting environment. Price (2013) highlighted the centrality of place in being human by stating that "human beings are not simply social animals; we are too spatial animals, inasmuch as territory—knowing it, owning it, exploring it—matters a great deal" (p. 119). In this respect, diversity is not a series of steps to take or a framework to master, rather it is an attitude, a detachment from the lexis of personal hubris to the gift of authentic encounter.

Practicing in place

When I enter the student research hub, I am enveloped by a sea of cubicles and the continuous clicking of keyboards. I walk past my cubicle and if I see my Mainland colleagues, we greet each other with a "Hi." Sometimes there is a smile and if one of us is near the entryway, we help open the door for the other. We share our research progress in the kitchenette and even provide consolation at times of immense grief, such as in the case of the support I received in the recent passing of my grandfather. In these small acts, there is an understanding beyond tolerance. Through this continued practice of engagement, relationships grow. In California, my comfort of being different was the feeling that everyone else was different around me too—that was the thread that connected us. The people and institutions surrounding me had celebrated difference positively, as though we all had something special to contribute.

Territorial transition was an 18th century memory unlike the current state of Hong Kong. I am thankful for being pushed into discomfort by my professor and group colleagues for I may have chosen group members holding value orientations similar to my own, defeating the purpose of being a PhD student in Hong Kong. In this new place, the residual complexities of a postcolonial territory absorbed into Greater China in conjunction with an unfolding political movement brought me to a completely different diversity experience. If I had retreated into the expatriate bubble of certainty, I would have robbed myself from the richness of difference that this place has to offer. Practicing in place allows me to walk into new life worlds and with every new encounter, I rediscover my place in diversity.

Note

1. The name *Ming* is a pseudonym in lieu of the real name of the group work member discussed in this article.

Reference

Price, P. (2013). Place. In N. Johnson, R. H. Schein, & J. Winders (Eds.), *The Wiley-Blackwell companion to cultural geography* (pp. 118–129). West Sussex, England: Wiley-Blackwell.

IN THE CLASSROOM

"The paradox of education is precisely this - that as one begins to become conscious one begins to examine the society in which [s]he is being educated."

James A. Baldwin

Being Black in a Higher Learning Institution

Destinee Miguest

This narrative portrays my experience as an African American woman in a predominantly White institution in which I feel diversity and inclusion are not sufficiently addressed or understood. I wrote this to encourage others who are a part of minority groups to continue to find their voices in this complex world.

Being black in a higher learning institution

It was my last semester of graduate school and I had survived the deathly verdicts of Michael Brown, Tamir Rice, Walter Scott, Eric Garner, and many other unarmed Black men living in the United States, who died at the hands of police over the course of 2 years. I use the term *survive* to emphasize the ignorance I experienced in the institution of higher education that I was attending.

Many may call my behavior as "flying under the radar," but I simply refer to it as "survival of the fittest." The rage I felt and grief I experienced, due to the loss of my brothers to senseless violence and policies based on melanin counts, went unspoken. My deep sensitivity to a system that works to protect the majority population, while perpetually challenging "the other," never seemed to hold the same importance as the topic of the day on the syllabus, even within a present context of serial killings by police of unarmed Black men.

My distress and fury had become my little secret. Whenever, my peers said something offensive, I never reacted. When my professors deducted points off pop quizzes with "constructive criticism" such as, "You didn't answer the question fully," without consideration that I may not have fully understood the questions due to a cultural barrier; I never reacted.

One of my degree qualifications was to take two group work courses: General and Substance Abuse focused. Both courses required students to participate in assigned groups picked by the professor. In my first group work course, the professor used a computer to randomly place students in two separate groups. One group was made up of all heterosexual White women ranging from early twenties to late fifties. The second group comprised nine heterosexual women in their twenties, one Asian and myself, an African American, and another African American woman who identified as homosexual.

I would describe the first group with high compatibility and low complexity. All members got along with ease, everyone participated, and everyone was engaged in the process. I would describe my group as having high compatibility and high complexity. We did not always get along, several members were consistently absent, and numerous members chose not to participate, indicating that their participation was not significant. I remember feeling so defeated after this experience. I think we truly had the potential to be a promising group. But with some believing that their participation was not important or, perhaps, not knowing how to interact with and embrace the diversity of a group like ours, the group floundered. I remember experiencing a familiar feeling of anger and rage. I didn't react. I just thought to myself, who do I talk to? Who can I trust with this secret? Little did I know, this experience would be repeated with a vengeance.

I took the next group work course 1 year later. The professor specified that he wanted to make sure the groups we would be assigned to would go into depth with the exercises he created. He created five small groups with approximately eight members in each. I ended up in a group with five White members, one Jewish, and one African American woman besides myself. This group presented with a more open and comfortable vibe, probably due to the fact that we previously had several classes together. However, even with a high level of comfort, the presence of diversity was a powerful force that affected the group's development.

I will never forget when diversity was the topic of discussion for the day. The majority of members in my group did not know their family histories and did not seem to care to know them. When it was my turn, I said that I identified as African American not Black. I explained it was because I knew my ancestors were from Africa, but that is all I know. Identifying as African American helps me to connect my roots and my identity.

If I had the opportunity to learn about my ancestors growing up in history class, maybe identity wouldn't be such a big deal. But for now, my identity reminds me that I am recognized as a half human being in the land of America. The response to what I shared was mostly blank stares from my peers and a couple of eyes ferociously holding back tears. One of the members in the group immediately reacted by endorsing that he hates being viewed as the bad guy by African Americans, "just for being White" and that all White people aren't bad." I didn't say anything else for the remainder of the group. Even though I know I did not offend that member, I was raised in a culture where it is crucial to be mature and understand why he felt the need to defend his race after I made the statement about my identity. That familiar feeling of rage surfaced and again/I thought at that moment, "Who do I talk to? Who can I trust with this secret?"

A few weeks later, the professor decided to combine all the groups for the exercise he planned that day. We were instructed to close our eyes and just listen with an open mind. He read this story about a fictitious world where everyone identified as homosexual. It was the norm, he said, and we listened.

We were raised in a family where our parents were homosexual; our older siblings were homosexual, as well as our friends. We were expected to go to prom with the same sex because it was what everyone else did. However, we were not homosexual. We were heterosexual but never said anything in fear of being kicked out of our homes, chastised/harassed by others who didn't understand, terminated from school, and more. So we kept this secret our entire lives, until we got to college. We went out one night and found a bar where everyone was heterosexual. It was the only one in town and not many homosexuals knew about it. We finally found a place where others shared our secret and understood exactly how we felt. Everyone shared heterosexual books and magazines that depicted similar experiences of other heterosexual people. We started going back week after week, because we developed a deep connection with these people that had never been felt before. One week, we met the love of our lives. We could only express this love in the bar though, and we agreed to keep this secret with our partners only. We dated for a couple years and knew we wanted to spend the rest of our lives together; but we couldn't get married. We couldn't even get an apartment together because landlords did not support heterosexual behavior. So we continued to meet at the bar, until one weekend, our partner didn't show up. We called but they never answered. We went to the bar again that next day, in hopes of seeing our other half again, but they never showed. We called them for a week straight but still there was no answer. We found out a couple weeks later from our homosexual friends that our partner had gotten into a car accident and died hours later in the hospital. We didn't get a chance to say good-bye because no one knew how special they were to us.

We held this secret and now all we could think was who do I talk to? Who can I trust with this secret?

The professor asked us to bring our attention back to the room. As hard as I tried, my tears would not cease. Although this exercise was an emotional one, I couldn't help but to feel triggered. The professor opened the floor for discussion and silence filled the room. One peer stated that she felt this was an example of oppression in general and that it could be applied to other "things," referring to other types of diversity and targets of oppression. The professor agreed but did not engage in that conversation. He simply reiterated that the floor was open for discussion. Several peers said how sad they felt and stated how deep this topic was. Finally, a heterosexual White woman stated, "I liked this exercise because it reminded me of how easily I can do things without having to think about it. It almost makes me feel bad in a sense." The professor responded by saying, "Yeah it's unfortunate, but don't beat yourself up about it, it's okay. This is not your fault."

I couldn't believe what I was hearing at that moment. Not only was I triggered, but now I felt defeated and unsupported by the most powerful individual in the room. The professor then asked if anyone had any other comments before we end class early. I debated in my mind for what felt like the longest minute of my life. I raised my hand and once I opened my mouth I couldn't stop. I explained how triggering this exercise was for someone like me who is a part of a minority group. Thus, it is crucial for the professor to remain neutral and support all variety of diversity in exercises like this. But, he failed to.

As soon as someone mentioned extending the meaning of this exercise to other oppressed groups, he minimized the significance of that comment. Not only that, when the White woman said the exercise reminded her of how easy it is for her to do things and how easily she forgets about the struggle of minority groups, he failed to encourage her not to be afraid to claim her White privilege in front of a "diverse" group.

The professor then took it a step further and defended her White privilege by dictating that she should not feel bad about forgetting she has it and then endorsing that it wasn't her fault. Although that may be true, I can easily argue the same thing. It isn't my fault that I am discriminated against, stereotyped, and undergo daily microaggressions by the majority population during my commute to and from school. I didn't choose oppression, it chose me. But the professor's White privilege didn't allow him to see that.

He is constantly validated in the world, from beauty, to education, to the law. Thus, whenever conversations like this one generate any discomfort for the majority population, surface-level comments become acceptable as a means to protect White privilege. But let me just say, it is "okay" to feel uncomfortable; and, it was the professor's job to push the discomfort everyone was experiencing at that moment to a deeper level.

I feel uncomfortable every single day, and the majority of people do not think twice about it. I should not have to live in a world where the majority population dictates when and where it is appropriate to converse about race and ethnicity based on their level of comfort.

I understand forgetting one's privilege is an easy thing to do, but every time my counterparts forget, they do nothing to help solve the issues of systemic oppression. Having White privilege does not make you a bad person. But often times, the majority population tends to associate it with racism, which they equate with a lack of moral values.

This is a type of dichotomous thinking pattern that our society has been socialized to practice since the Civil Rights Movement. Oppression has always been more than just Black and White thinking. Race is on a spectrum that includes other oppressive classifications such as sexuality, class, gender, and more. Surviving isn't enough for me anymore. For me to live freely, we need groups like the ones that I just described to start addressing and celebrating the true nature and importance of diversity across the entire spectrums, instead of endlessly debating who's at fault for the lack of progress of minority groups. And maybe then, the answer to my questions, "who do I talk to? who can I trust?" will begin to be answered.

Until the Animals Get Their Own Story Teller, the Hunter Remains the Hero of All Tales

Olufunke Oba

I keep quiet, even though every fiber of me feels like screaming. An outburst from me would only reinforce notions of the angry Black woman. Jan, Madeline, and Vanessa carry on without missing a beat. I sit there sweaty and speechless as the turmoil rages within me. The cacophony of voices drowns out all but their own. I cannot believe that they think they can decide everything in the first meeting: the topic, the format, and the tasks for our group presentation. I am stunned. But I remain silent. They actually suggested that my task would be to help them change the slides, set up the room, and arrange snacks for the class. As morning dawns and night fades, so does my dream as reality introduces itself anew.

I find myself retreating deeper and deeper into my seat, feeling small, and wanting to just drop down dead. They act nice when they tell me they don't want to put me through the speaking part as it can be challenging for those who are not used to it. But I feel silenced, angry, hurt, humiliated, and small. Where is my voice? Where is my agency? I seek words and find none. I wonder: Can there be agency without voice? Why do they assume that presenting before the class would be hard for me and not for them? What does this say about what they think of me?

The academy seeks diversity but doesn't seem prepared for it. Is it any surprise that people of diversity do not feel as if they fit in these places? The realities of race and place are complex. Why would Black students apply? Here I am. I was accepted into graduate school fair and square, but do my peers know that? Do they believe it?

I am in a group with three women who appear to be friends and one man. The women have decided that only their ideas are likely to earn the group a good grade. What's more, they have predetermined who can give good presentations. We learn that Jan's father works as a psychologist at the local hospital. Jan says that our adapting the hospital's model for a different population would give us an advantage.

My palms are sweaty, my tongue clings to my dry throat, and my heart pounds. I wonder if the group can hear my loud breathing. But I need not

---

Adapted from an African proverb

worry because I am invisible to them. Invisibility provides reprieve from the White gaze, but I cannot be invisible forever. What I really want is to be seen for who I am as opposed to being dismissed and assigned to set up the room and arrange for snacks.

Despite all of the diversity rhetoric, my Black body is missing. We talk of postcolonialism, but certain types of knowledge are invalidated. My insides churn, but it does not seem to matter. Although absented, my Black body is very visible. Yet my voice is closeted because it does not fit the hegemonic discourse. Gripped by fear, I long to escape. Maybe someone will say something. Instead they pack up and make their way out together, leaving me in a daze.

The abyss of colonization

I am not alone, there are two of us just sitting, bewildered and wondering what just happened. He looks my way, I try to catch his gaze, and he drops his face, mumbling inaudibly as he shuffles uncomfortably. Alan says he's in the part-time program as he cannot afford to study full time. My elation about returning to school and the hope it represented to me, and anticipated sense of belonging, is already eroding.

In anticipation of my return to school, I fantasized about long debates and grappling with tensions and complexities. I was euphoric envisioning what an elite tribe of scholars can accomplish. The critical thinking and discourses that I imagined do not materialize. Smiling faces make my acquaintance, but the university is just another site of colonization. My broken self realizes that social justice and diversity are little more than noble ideas in this place.

The academy delegitimizes experiential knowledge garnered from the school of life. Stories and proverbs are disdained as folklore. Reciprocity, communality, and mutuality are hallmarks of traditions in indigenous communities across the globe. What better place for such traditions to be celebrated than in group work.

Nevertheless, I feel as if I don't exist here. But my shaking hands and racing heart tell me I do. I am alive and well, but how shall I choose to exist. Do I acquiesce or transgress? Shall I accept the barriers and structures that exclude indigenous knowledge or resist? In the evening I imagine the conversations that they must have in the privacy of their homes as I converse with no one, but myself, and steel myself for a better tomorrow.

Resolving to transgress

Our grades are important, but so are the people whose lives we will hold in our hands as we intervene with youths, survivors of war, refugees, and others. I know I can't keep silent. I feel anguish. My Black body has access, but what I embody is disdained and to speak is to mark myself. I continue to inhabit marginal spaces like fellow Blacks inside and outside of the academy. Tears, groans, and prayers spoken or unexpressed are my companions on this lonely journey. I speak not of myself but of all Black people. Antioppression without action hinders the healing and transformative potential of group work.

> How do I emplace me in this space?
> All of me, spirit, soul, body and voice, in this place
> When parts of me are unwelcome in this space?
> Can the whole of me and the self that is whole be present?
> I seek to be alive, reflected, and represented in the school's tenet
> For the sake of the marginalized and vulnerable absent here
> Who are harmed or helped daily by what social workers learn here
> I make up my mind; I will not lose my mind
> To see the change, I must be the change
> Love finds a way, makes one where others cringe.

I do not want to be called a whiner or poor team player. Feminists, postracial scholars, and critical thinkers flock the halls, but do they understand? Multicultural rhetoric, use of self, cultural competency, and tolerance are professed, but is tolerance acceptance? Cultural competency that is not about self-mastery disavows the lived reality of "the other." My ideas gather dust and my brain goes to rust. I must escape this bleak night of the soul by pushing through this dark hole. And so with much trepidation, I send off this group e-mail to my group, for the sake of all the marginalized people out there.

> Hi group,
> Thanks to the ladies for coordinating the meeting today; it was obvious you came prepared with awesome ideas and plans for our group, but I feel other ideas were ignored and to avoid lurking resentment, I think it is important for everyone to have their say.
> I really appreciate your passion and push for all of us to get good grades. Trust me; I want that too, but preoccupation with grades that makes us forget why we are here or why we wanted to be social workers in the first place does not feel right. Ignoring process and group dynamics can cost us grades and much more. Remember the group stages? We don't want to set ourselves up for a major storm, but beyond that what of our clients?
> Could I suggest we reconvene for an icebreaker and brainstorming session? We are a very strong team with strengths, and lots of life and work experiences so we can pull off the grades, but please, let's do it together as a group and as future group facilitators.
> I look forward to working with you all, thanks for your time and consideration.
> Funke

Was it respectful enough? What will they think of me? They already think I am dragging the group down bringing Afrocentric ideas into the group. They'll want nothing to do with me and I will have to change groups. I hate begging to join groups, it transports me right back to the elementary school yard.

Self-doubt arises as I toss and turn, fearing the worst. I feel as if I am judged incapable because I believe in indigenous, spiritual, and intuitive ways of understanding life's complex phenomena. School is becoming intense but not because of what it is giving me but what it wants to wrest from me. A paternalistic, patronizing, hierarchy of knowledge denigrates my oral traditions and spiritual knowledge.

Afrocentricism as a framework for group work

The moment of reckoning is here. It's the group's first meeting after my e-mail.

There is no backing out now, I will not self-censure or curl up and snore. We are all polite, but it is awkward. Alan and I sit on one side while Jan, Madeline, and Vanessa sit at another table. Still, we begin with a game to get to know one another better and actually have fun. We have many "aha" moments as we discover commonalities such as pets, hobbies, vacations, and favorite ice-cream toppings.

After the ice-breaker games, we proceed to hear everyone's ideas. Jan recaps the ideas presented by Madeline, Vanessa, and her at the first meeting. I am called upon to go next and speak about Afrocentric group work and its effectiveness for addressing mental health, trauma, social skills, and anger management. I talk about what it can afford clinicians and group facilitators with respect to true antioppressive work and mutual empowerment. I add that it is well suited to working with Black males and marginalized youth generally because its participatory features such as movement and art compliment traditional talk therapy.

I explain, for example, that drumming can be a release and dance as a form of exercise can help people to relax and feel comfortable enough to let out deep feelings and emotions. Rhythm, pacing, coordination of hands and hearts also enhance impulse control whereas social connections, cultural pride, and stimulation of un-accessed parts of the brain can produce overall mental, emotional, and physical health.

I go on to explain that African healing forms represented in music, rap, or stories start from the known to the unknown, taking the person-in-context approach, and can therefore resonate with and engage Africans. By combining features of intergenerational oral traditions, physical and music therapy, Afrocentric groups can harness the verbal, nonverbal, mental, and emotional. I go on to say that it can break down barriers and reduce distance between experts and those who are socially constructed as nonknowers. Singing, clapping, dancing, and drumming promote connections among people who may never have thought they have anything in common.

Group work can promote self-discovery as group members learn and mirror one another's journey and support one another in the safety of the group. This is an evolving area that is particularly relevant as Canada becomes more and more diverse and the population of Africans and other minority groups increase rapidly due to liberalization of race-based immigration regulations. Modelling this innovative approach and coaching peers to use it with diverse clients can contribute to decolonized therapies gaining recognition in the academy.

A journey in integration

There it was. I had said what needed to be said. We were going around the table to hear everyone's perspectives. It was Alan's turn to speak. To my surprise, he starts clapping and the others join in. I see a new found admiration written all over their faces. Alan insists he really wants to learn about this emergent therapy, adding that in his agency they regularly see African families, refugees, and international students with amazing strengths. He notes that traditional deficit-based interventions don't work for them, so this would be great learning.

One by one, the others echo his words, saying they love it. I am shocked by their enthusiasm. Their energy is palpable, but I shy away from carrying the responsibility for the group's fate in my hands. Then I remember a Nigerian proverb that says "until the animals get their own story teller, the hunter remains the hero of all tales." There is no doubt in my mind that if I take leadership my Black body will be under surveillance. But I am encouraged with the knowledge that restorative justice, kinship family systems, and other communal approaches have been similarly integrated into the mainstream. I remind the group that many of the steps are undocumented and that we would all have to work very hard together as I am no expert and have no ready-made manuals. We go around and each member commits to the tasks of integrating Afrocentric and Eurocentric worldviews in group work.

All I ever wanted was to be heard, I can't believe we're going out on a limb together. We designed a 12-week group utilizing stories, proverbs, art, and dance. Jan and Vanessa choreographed the dance after watching YouTube videos. Madeline and I created the slides, and Alan devised an evaluation that was visual and based on African agriculture. Crops represented wholesome thoughts and habits while weeds stood for things to be uprooted. This tool enabled us to identify systemic and individual components of the soil in people's lives. The response to our presentation was overwhelmingly positive, everyone had fun dancing and the ripple effects included other groups wanting me on their teams and invitations to present in other classes.

Group debriefing

Jan said she'd been seriously thinking about her preoccupation with grades and the pressure of living up to the expectations of her psychologist father as he not only wanted her to get a job in the hospital but also to join his private practice. She said this group helped her see the need to follow her passions. We all reflected on how this project challenged us, exposed our biases, and caused us to grow as persons. Alan opened up about messages of inadequacy he received from his mother as a child and how that was triggered in the group. He said listening to Jan showed him that everyone has a story. Madeline said she always assumed men have all the power. Vanessa said coming from a small Newfoundland community she had never had any experience interacting with Black people. She helped me see similarities in the stereotyping of Africans and Newfoundlanders. She said this group was the best thing to happen to her as it challenged her to learn not just theories but to engage in self-discovery and experiential learning.

On my part, the insights I gained from this group will enhance my ability to continue to mentor Black youths who are marginalized in the school system. I had to practice what I teach by taking the risk for my own learning. By placing a premium on my knowledge, I enabled others to respect what I had. People who are plagued by their own insecurities may not easily embrace others, but this group together surmounted our varied anxieties and successfully counteracted entrenched and previously unexamined notions of Eurocentric universality.

I know I may not be able to change the world, but addressing microaggressions and reshaping group dynamics transparently, and gently, "in here" can affect the work we do "out there." It is not enough that things happen to us, it is important that we reflect on them to make meaning of the experience and grow. Sharing my group's success, lifelong friendships, and the opportunities it afforded us can hopefully change habitual orientations to diverse students in the academy. As a group, through tear-filled eyes as we shared a warm group hug, we concluded that we would never again see group work the same way.

Recognizing the Needs of Black Social Work Students in the Current Racial Climate

Norissa J. Williams

One Friday night in the fall semester of 2014 I was presenting a lecture in the social work course Child Welfare. It was my first semester at Medgar Evers College, a junior college within the City University of New York. As a historically Black College with its mission is rooted in the ideals of its namesake and a location in Central Brooklyn, it is primarily attended by people of African descent.

Prior to Medgar Evers I had taught for 5 years and presented a number of trainings in the community. This was the first time I had taught in an all-Black setting. In other mixed-race but predominantly White classroom settings where I taught, issues of race didn't come up as much. It wasn't the central organizing principle in how these individuals related to the world and the how the world related to them—a luxury not easily afforded by people of color.

Another significant difference between the classes I was now teaching and those I had taught before was the fact that we were living in a different racial climate. Things had changed in a very short period of time.

Trayvon Martin

In February 2012 Trayvon Martin, a 17-year-old African American boy was walking home from a convenience store in Miami, Florida after purchasing candy and a drink. He was wearing a hooded black sweater when George Zimmerman, a neighborhood watch volunteer, saw him. Zimmerman perceived him to be a threat and called police. Even though Zimmerman was warned not to approach Martin, he did. A fight ensued and Zimmerman killed an unarmed Martin, claiming self-defense.

Zimmerman was not immediately arrested. Many believed the response would have been different if a White teen had been killed. Moreover, many believed that Martin was stereotyped and perceived to be a threat simply because he was Black. When Zimmerman was arrested and the case eventually brought to trial in 2013, a jury of six women found Zimmerman not guilty in the shooting death of Trayvon Martin. Despite many people believing that the problem of racial profiling was at play in this case, there was still a large portion of America who believed that race had nothing to do with it.

For many, this was viewed as a single incident that could be argued away as "isolated." I wasted little time in my classes engaging students in discussions about how unconscious bias does in fact influence perception and action. I also shared personal experiences of being a target of racist behavior. Issues of race would soon reach a tipping point as a result of increased media coverage and social media chatter regarding incidents pertaining to the disproportionate and excessive use of force by police on black people.

Eric Garner

In July 2014, Eric Garner, a 43-year-old father of six and a New York City resident, was believed to be illegally selling loose cigarettes on a street corner in Staten Island. When Mr. Garner was approached by police he denied the allegation and stated that he was tired of being harassed. A police officer then tried to arrest him. Garner swatted the policeman away. The police officer then jumped on his back and wrapped his arm around Garner's neck in what many believed to be an illegal chokehold, ultimately bringing Garner to the pavement. While being choked he said repeatedly that he couldn't breathe. This was captured on a cell phone video taken by a bystander. The video went viral for the whole world to see and hear Mr. Garner pleading, "I can't breathe" 11 times, and then he stopped making noise. He was declared dead when he arrived to the hospital an hour later. Medical examiners declared it a homicide. The police officer who applied the chokehold went before a grand jury. They declined to indict him.

The students I taught at that time could identify with Trayvon Martin— innocently wearing hoodies, uninvolved in any criminal activity, and yet still treated suspiciously. They could also identify with Eric Garner who believed he was being harassed on a regular basis by virtue of his skin color. They each had their own personal stories. When they weren't the subject of harassment, their brothers, cousins, fathers, husbands or boyfriends were. The national media coverage of these events led many of my students, and many Black people nationwide, to vicariously experience a level of trauma that demanded attention. Needing catharsis, the issue of race came up more and more in class—even in classes as seemingly remote as Research Methods.

My student

One evening, a student shared that earlier that day on his way to school, he was entering the train station with a book bag on his back. A police officer stopped him, asking to search his book bag. He felt that he hadn't done anything to warrant such suspicion and being the radical individual that he is, he said, "No." He resisted the controversial "Stop and Frisk" command that had been criticized by many New Yorkers as legalized racial profiling. He told them that he knew his rights and wouldn't let them be violated. Consequently he was denied entrance on the train and had to take a taxi to school instead.

My dilemma

I was (and still am) proud of this student for standing up for something he believed in. He was courageous in a way many would not have been—resisting being demeaned by what he deemed a racist practice. But, the other part of me begged, "Stop! No! Don't do that again…" with silent whispers of, "I want you to live." This fear and conformity was uncharacteristic of me, but in this moment it had become me. I was afraid for his life, and the life of all those whose hue resembled his—including my own son. As the moderator of the discussion, students looked to me, their "knowledgeable" professor, for an answer. Was that the right response? Is that how one brings about social change—resisting individually? Should a more passive approach be adopted?

I opened the floor waiting to hear the opinion of others because I really didn't know what to say. I was feeling a sense of fear and paralysis that I didn't recognize. Had I not been the mother of a Black boy, my advice would have been different. I would have easily said the student had done the right thing. Statistics were showing that Black and brown men were disproportionately targeted and this felt like more of the same. However, when I thought about my son and the fact that something like that could end in death, I thought, "Just do what they say and live … put your hands up. Yes, sir. No ma'am. Here's my book bag. Whatever you have to do, just do it." The problem with the latter thought is how demeaning it feels.

Recently, as I drove to work I saw a police car pull over a caravan. A Black man was driving. Immediately, after pulling over safely, I saw the man stick his two hands out of the window, as if to urgently assert that, "I'm not armed! Please, don't shoot!" It's difficult to put into words, but it bothers me deeply that this is what a Black man feels he has to do to increase his chances of living. I drove by sadly, wondering what this fear was doing collectively to the psyche of this country. I reflected back on the classroom discussion that Friday night. The same radical student who refused to turn over his book bag said that the current state of fear that Black people in America are experiencing is reminiscent of the fear experienced when the Ku Klux Klan was active in the deep south and mothers and wives urged their spouses and children to get home before it was dark, for fear of lynching. Such memories have a way of reviving old and deep psychic wounds in the same the way loud noises can cause former soldiers suffering from posttraumatic stress to have flashbacks and relive former traumatic events.

Tilting sideways in a slanted room

Assuming a position of surrender in a situation that should (at maximum) only require you to pull over is not only demeaning, it's problematic. It's like tilting sideways in a slanted room to accommodate the distortion, leading everyone to believe that you're standing straight (Harris-Perry, 2011). It is conforming as opposed to standing up to a flawed and toxic environment in need of repair. Given this view, I wondered how could I rightly encourage my students to lose themselves in resignation, knowing what this has done psychologically in generations past in America. The dilemma is obvious. I recognized that I couldn't encourage such resignation, but I also couldn't encourage them to resist in the way my brave student had. I wouldn't be able to live with myself, if on my word they resisted and ultimately lost their life. But what happens to social workers if we teach our students and supervisees to be satisfied with the status quo?

The emotional state of my students

The conversation that Friday night was one of many similar ones during that semester. My students' asking eyes spoke to the emotional state of Black youth and their families all over America. They had the fortunate advantage of being in an environment where they were not the minority but could use the class and the college itself as a means to grow through this period in American history. They were not hushed, nor were their thoughts dismissed as mine had been so many times in contexts where I was the sole Black person in the room. For that I was happy. Yet these emerging social workers—whether spoken or unspoken—experienced a level of fear that caused them to socialize their children, younger siblings, and male family members in ways that they had not previously done. Their anger led them to want to do something greater to affect change. What they wanted was for those who were to come after them to have better lives, in the same way they benefited from the activist work of the civil rights movement of their parents' and grandparents' generation. The unfortunate sense of hopelessness that concluded a number of our conversations has motivated me to do more. It reminded me of why I became a social worker.

Conclusion

I wish I could say that since 2014 things have changed in the country. However, there have been even more race related incidents. In April 2015 Freddie Gray, a 25-year-old black man died in police custody after being arrested for possession of an illegal switchblade. This incident led to civil unrest and rioting in the city of Baltimore, Maryland. In April 2015, Walter Scott, an unarmed Black man in South Carolina was killed by police, shot in the back, after being pulled over for a nonfunctioning brake light. In June 2015 Black youths were captured on a cell phone camera being treated roughly and unfairly at a pool incident in McKinney, Texas. And, at the time of this writing we are only 2 weeks shy of the horrific Charleston, North Carolina, church shooting in which nine unarmed people were murdered by a 21-year-old White man who said he wanted to start a race war.

This country is in a state of crisis and flux with respect to race relations. America finds itself again at a tipping point that hearkens back to the civil rights movement of the 1960s. It is time for the next generation of leaders to emerge and find their place in confronting a disdainful past (and present) that is supported by institutionalized racism.

Social work students may just be the ones to lead the way. However, when we are with our groups of students of all shades and hues it is important to note that they are more than our future leaders and potential saviors and that they have emotional needs. Let's not lose sight of the fact that the needs of Black and brown students may be more complex than we realize.

As a teacher and person of color and mother of a Black boy, I know that my students at Medgar Evers College are vulnerable. Medgar Evers was a civil rights activist who worked to overturn segregation at the University of Mississippi in the 1960s. A World War II veteran, Evers was later assassinated for his activism.

When I see my students sitting before me, I struggle every day with striking a balance between encouraging them to stand up and lead the way and stand down to save their lives.

Reference

Harris-Perry, M. V. (2011). *Sister citizen: Shame, stereotypes, and black women in America.* New Haven, CT: Yale University Press.

Flowers and a Garden, Children and Games, Laughter and Fun: Unity in Diversity

Reineth Prinsloo, Jenilee Botha, Lee-Ann Human, Lindokuhle Maphalala, Thato Masuku, Zipho Tshapela, and Evadné van den Berg

Social work declares its commitment to respect and valuing human dignity, to acceptance, unconditional positive regard, equity, self-determination, a nonjudgmental approach and social justice. When I, as group work professor, entered the 3rd year social work class at the beginning of this year (2015), it was disturbing to see the way that the students divided themselves with regard to culture, language, and even age to some extent. After providing an orientation about the content of the module on advanced group work skills, I reflected on what I observed and confronted the students. Being dedicated to teaching sensitivity to diversity, I told the students that I refuse to teach a senior social work student group that is divided and where students do not mingle, bond, and integrate.

Consequently, I arranged for a 3-hour experiential class the next week, to be held on the university's sports grounds close to our main campus. The aim of the class was to be twofold: first, to let the students experience being group members, and second, to address the issues of division that I observed. Not only should group workers help members to recognize differences and understand them, they should also recognize and understand their own values and differences. Group workers' worldviews, beliefs, and values of group influence their practice. I feel strongly about the fact that a social worker, and especially a group worker, has to be aware of his or her own values and perceptions before attempting to engage with others.

The activities that I planned aimed at providing fun and relaxation yet providing a deep focus on integration of theory and becoming aware of each other. Students had to play with soccer balls, dance to the rhythm of music, do team activities (in united fashion), such as picking up hula hoops and passing them without breaking a circle held together by holding hands. They played games from their childhood years and had to teach each other these childhood games. I wanted to take them back to being a child: the place where we are socialized and where family of origin and childhood contexts form current perspectives, values, and beliefs.

I witnessed an amazing transformation. Before they realized what was happening, they were asking each other about the origin of the games and were starting to repeat the instructions in each other's mother tongues, even if pronounced awkwardly. They laughed and I had to ask one of the students who could whistle loudly to get their attention to continue to another exercise. The atmosphere was one of pure bliss! Students who never before communicated did so now. Seventy students danced in harmony as one long train to the songs of different cultural groups.

The last exercise for the day was completing the 3rd-year group work class garden on a huge poster. Two students assisted me prior to the class to paint a basic garden with two prominent trees. Every student present at the experiential class had to paint his or her own flower in the garden. They had a choice of paintbrushes and different colors of paint. I commented that the poster painting formed one garden, yet not two of the flowers were the same. The unity in diversity made for one beautiful and color-filled garden in which the students, who were divided before the class commenced, departed as one large bonded group. The feedback was amazing. The stories that follow provide a view of the transformation that transpired on that glorious day, from the perspective of six students.

Reflections

Jenilee: Nacre is my answer

Nacre is my answer. "The answer to what?" one might ask, thereupon I shall elaborate with the utmost of confidence, "the answer to most problems in society!" Group work has proven itself to me in so many ways before and after, but on this specific occasion, I was gleefully aware of how it feels to be a part of the problem, and part of the solution; and as nacre believe, a part of something beautiful.

Nacre is the calcium carbonate layer of silky, luminous, and iridescent substance lined on the inside of a pearl-producing oyster. As it happens in nature, as well as in our daily lives, many conflicts arise from the fear of "something different." When a grain of sand finds its way through the clasps of an oyster, it moves to stay on the bedded cushion in the middle of the organism where it then causes a discomfort. This strange object is perceived as a threat, and in the process of protecting itself, the oyster will continuously cover the grain of sand with a special substance made out of millions of light-reflecting particles. This substance is called nacre and will be layered over the grain of sand many times until it hardens, which then forms what we know to be as a beautifully valuable pearl.

In my experience, group work is precisely described through this miraculous process that nature has created to turn something problematic into something extraordinary. On this specific occasion, diversity within our class was acting as the grain of sand that has made its way into the hearts of the class members. Differences in culture, appearance, and even language created an environment of fear and discomfort. Nationwide, and South Africa in specific, countries have vast varieties of ethnicities, cultural backgrounds, and religions, which have managed to become a threat to large populations of its inhabitants. This was the students' experience, even within a class dedicated to enhancing equality and acceptance among all people.

However, because of group work and the uplifting participation in one glorious morning of genuine *Ubuntu* (an ancient African word meaning "humanity to others"), the discomfort and fear of everything different was challenged and turned into a beautiful product. As with an oyster, the classroom members were exposed to the worlds of others through working together, mutual sharing. and going back to the fun activities of youth. The beauty in each culture was found by all, generating layers and layers of team work until the product was a class full of members with respect for one another and for diversity, as if a precious pearl.

In this world of shifting sands, group work as we experienced it on that morning, was at the heart of a beautiful nacre world.

Lindokuhle: I was no longer standing on my own guarding a tree

There is absolutely nothing more frustrating to a student than the words *compulsory attendance*. We try to avoid taking a shower, dressing up, and coming to campus and interacting with people. One can only then imagine the feeling when Professor Prinsloo informed us that she had planned a joint group activity for our entire class. I try to avoid group activities; I always stick out like a sore thumb or cling to the one person who was brave enough to talk to me first.

I have always known Professor Prinsloo to be an energetic and an inspirational lecturer. However, I did feel that this time she was just pushing things way too far. I honestly felt race and diversity and unity will always be an issue regardless of the many times we try to address it. I always felt it should rather be swept under the carpet and that nobody should talk about it.

The day of our joint class activity came and, as usual, being the social butterfly that she is, my only friend left me standing in the middle of a crowd. Which was really awkward because these are the same people I have attended class with for the past 3 years and you would think by now we would have gotten to know each other? As I was standing there, I noticed that everyone was clustered in little groups of their close circle of friends until Professor Prinsloo scattered us around and formed us into different groups. We all stood in awe; giving each other awkward little smiles as we listened to Professor giving us activity instructions.

It was only at the end of our group exercise that I realized the group dynamics that took place during the activities, including the importance of communication, the emergence of a group leader, and the development of group norms.

I also realized that I was no longer standing on my own guarding a tree but together mingling with my classmates and playing games we used to play when we were young. Even if you did not understand the game, you would just join in and make a complete fool of yourself and you will catch the rules of the game as you play. It was also fun to play games from the other races (cultural groups) as well. We mumbled some of the Afrikaans recitals, but we continued playing. Not only was it fun but a wonderful experience seeing some of the White students joining in and trying to figure out all the dance moves.

It didn't matter, then, who you were standing next to or holding hands with or looking out for a familiar face to throw a ball to, because it was "at that moment" that we were united. We were not forced to get along, we could have chosen to remain in our little shells and comply with whatever Professor had planned for us. The great part in all of this was that it expanded our knowledge and our insight on the little differences we have that we sometimes then choose to turn into big deals.

The memory of this wonderful day that opened up the children in us lives on the 10th floor of the Human Science Building.

Evadnè: What I saw was magical!

Spring has always brought wonder to me, and every year I still stand in awe of how the dullness of winter seems to disappear within the blink of an eye when the flowers start to bloom. With age the realization came that flowers do not magically bloom when fairies sprinkle their pixie dust over the flower buds; it is a process that requires time, the right environment, and the correct climate.

I have found this wonderfully intricate process can be compared to the awareness and acceptance of diversity, and how a garden is formed by putting together different flowers; all of them beautiful in their own way. One flower does not think of competing with the one next to it, it just blooms. This year I had the privilege to see how the magical process of the coming of spring happened within our group work class.

When thinking back to before our experiential class the interaction between our students sometimes seemed to be like winter in a way, dull and cold. My metaphor might sound a bit harsh, but I have always found that I experience things in extremes and the lack of communication and division among students in our class broke my heart. I guess this was partially due to my belief that one can love and accept all human beings and that we are not defined by the color of our skin, but rather the condition of our hearts. In everything I do I strive to love people for their hearts, and not for their characteristics or circumstances. This notion has left me speechless, confused, and disappointed many times.

One of the exercises during our experiential class was that of creating our own garden. This was an arts and crafts activity where each student had the opportunity to paint a flower on a poster, under the shade of two symbolic trees that formed a heart. During this exercise, I had the task of assisting the other students with the paintbrushes and paint. It offered me the opportunity to observe the interaction between them while painting. What I saw was magical!

I was in awe with how the students started to communicate with each other. For a moment it seemed like they were playing Twister, seeing how their arms intertwined, creating a space for everyone to paint their flowers. It was just as wonderful to see students who usually do not talk, laugh, and complement each other on the flowers that they have painted, with numerous students also helping each other with ideas and advice on how and where to paint their flowers.

I believe that this activity and the other activities from the experiential class bonded the students, giving us the much-needed opportunity to "find" one another, leading to the realization that we were not as different as we thought we were. Every time I look at the poster of our garden or walk past it in the corridor, I remember the day spring arrived in our class and when the flowers started to bloom.

Zipho: Previously I thought group work was about sitting and talking

From my perspective, group work practice has always been one-sided, monotonous, and uninteresting. However, the experience in the garden changed my perspective for the better. We discovered that group work can be enjoyable and that the best way to understand diversity is not only by talking about it but by having some fun while learning.

Previously I thought that group work was about sitting and talking about a certain topic, but the garden experience opened my eyes. Physical activities are very effective, relaxing, and refreshing; they allow group members to get to know each other in a pleasant atmosphere. After that day, I told myself that this is how I would like my group members to feel after group work sessions with me.

Besides being fun, the activities that we did were also challenging. For example, in the first activity we had to work together as a group to lift up a "hula hoop" and bring it down. It seemed like a very simple activity, but when it came to the execution, it became tricky. Within the group there were different genders and personalities; some wanted the activity to be done quick, some were too slow, a number of individuals wanted to lead and others were passive. Although this level of diversity made things complicated, it still helped us to adjust and be flexible with people who were different from ourselves.

In addition, the other activities of the day also highlighted the presence of diversity in race and culture. I learned new songs, new games, and new dance moves, which was very exciting. As much as there were differences, there were similarities as well. I learned that it is helpful to have some similarities when composing a group. I realized how our similarities brought us together because there was a sense of sharing common ground.

Lee-Ann: A person is a person because of people

Desmond Tutu once said,

> A person is a person through other persons. None of us comes into the world fully formed. We would not know how to think, or walk, or speak, or behave as human beings unless we learned it from other human beings. We need other human beings in order to be human. I am because other people are. A person is entitled to a stable community life, and the first of these communities is the family. ("Desmond Tutu," 2015)

Tutu's words of wisdom were summarized in the Zulu proverb: *Umuntu Ngumuntu Ngabantu* ("A person is a person because of people").

My fellow students and I had difficulty grasping the full essence of the message in the beginning, but after the experiential learning class we understood the proverb. It was interesting to see, once we started participating in numerous group activities, how we started to laugh, sing, dance, and cry in the same language. We were no longer separated by race, language, or gender. We became equal and they became one. There was one specific activity that we participated in, that is still one of my fondest memories today, it was called "There is a fire in the mountain."

We were asked to make groups of four, five, 10, and even 20 people. We then had to run and grab hold of one another to form these groups. Without hesitation we started to run toward one another without thinking about race, gender, or home language for 1 second. Not only did we gather more knowledge about different activities we can use during group work interventions but we also acquired the ability to communicate in one language without barriers. I remember looking around at my fellow classmates noticing that not one student was without a smile.

The activities were filled with 3rd-year social work students laughing, playing, and getting to know one another better. Previously in the classroom, the students were fairly disconnected from one another, but on that specific day, Professor Prinsloo made it possible for us to connect with one another regardless of our race, home language, or gender. I recall that the activities required us to listen to each other, work together, and to encourage one another when we were completing group activities.

On that day I gained a lot of respect for my fellow classmates and realized that we should all be working together to make the world a better place. I now understand the importance of embracing the uniqueness of each individual. Yes, diversity is what makes us different, but diversity can help us look at the problem from different perspectives, which will help us to intervene in the best possible way to empower our clients and motivate change.

On that day I became a different person. Although I started the day filled with my own perspectives and ideas, I finished the day as a person who recognized the importance of diversity, along with the uniqueness of each individual. Experiential learning creates the opportunity for us to see that group work interventions can be enjoyable and fun and can help to eliminate barriers between fellow group members.

Thato: I felt a certain level of closeness to my classmates

Socialization groups help members learn how to get along and do what is socially acceptable while educational groups help members learn new information and skills. Socialization and educational groups are used in a variety of settings including treatment agencies and schools.

On this particular day we, as students, were part of a socialization group that was also educational. The purpose of this team-building day was to equip us with new information and skills about how to approach group work as a treatment method in social work, at the same time we get to know each other. Part of the purpose of both types of groups is to address needs and challenges faced by group members.

During the past 2 years, I attended class with people I did not see as possible friends but only colleagues. I felt excluded, bored, and alone most of the time in class. This was because I thought I was older than the classmates were and had been at the university longer than most of them. This resulted in me feeling that I had nothing in common with them and could not form friendships with them. I saw them as colleagues and people I went to class with only.

The group work team-building day was a very fun, educative, and eye-opening experience for me. We had so much fun working together to accomplish goals. While executing the activities planned for the day, I learned about the similarities between my colleagues, their personalities, and the type of people they are (as well as myself). I made new friends among the group members (classmates).

This experience changed not only the way I view my classmates but also the manner in which I approach learning as a whole. After the team-building day, I felt a certain level of closeness to my classmates. This experience also improved the way I approach group work with my group members at CR Swart high school. It gave me new and innovative ideas of how I can help and make my group work fun and enjoyable and benefiting the groups I work with socially and emotionally.

During one of the activities we were asked to draw ourselves as flowers in the garden. I realized how unique each flower was, expressing its different qualities and characteristics that make it beautiful through art and color. This represented how unique and diverse we are as students. The garden contributes to our development by giving us necessary nutrients to make sure we grow to be beautiful flowers. Together as flowers, our uniqueness (different characteristics and contributions to this garden) make this garden look extremely beautiful.

We became closer to each other, learned to accept and respect each other's differences and uniqueness, cultures, and beliefs. We also became close by learning about the practices and games that influenced our ways of life. We helped each other to achieve tasks through communicating and learning about our roles in the group. Group work can be fun while we learn!

Conclusion

The universe is unique;, the world is filled with differences, minds think in different ways, colors split us, languages separate us, history divides us. Yet coming together and bridging divides bring sunshine and smiles and acceptance. This experiential class aimed to bring a divided group of senior social work students together. The class aimed at a concrete experience of what it means to be a group member and to experience the dynamic process of becoming one group, regardless of individual differences. Would the key to addressing judgment and discrimination be planned exercises where people be taken back to childhood, fun, laughter, and games? And then continuously reflecting on what is happening? My answer to this is: Yes! Not only have I witnessed transformation but the students reflected in their feedback how they became one unit, yet did not lose any of their individual characteristics and uniqueness.

Everyone smiles in the same language. (Unknown)

Reference

Desmond Tutu. (2015). Retrieved from https://www.goodreads.com/author/quotes/5943. Desmond_Tutu

Countertransference Challenges in Working with Diversity: A Group Worker Reflects

Les Fleischer

As a child of a holocaust survivor, I always recognized that diversity is an important topic in clinical practice, and a loaded issue for me personally. Prejudice, racism, and discrimination can cause great emotional pain, can result in murder and the attempted annihilation of entire groups or nations. So I thought that my self-awareness would counter any tendency I might have to aversely respond to clients who express anti-Semitic views, or other prejudices. However, this idea was challenged when I realized I forgot to attend a regularly scheduled appointment with a client who had recently been conveying anti-Semitic views.

A pleasant stroll

Instead of meeting him for his regularly scheduled appointment, I went for a pleasant stroll, oblivious to the fact that my client was waiting for me, and I only learned that I had missed the appointment when he left me an angry phone message, asking, "What happened?" Upon reflecting on my slip, I realized that I was much angrier than I had recognized. I had mostly pushed these thoughts and feelings away, aware that I was irritated, but I failed to recognize how much his comments had affected me. So, instead of acting on the (preconscious) urge to throw him out of my office, I removed myself, and essentially accomplished the same thing!

This experience highlighted the extent to which our own reactions (countertransference) can negatively affect our ability to effectively manage clients' prejudice. I reflected on how these difficulties may be exacerbated in group work, in which we must potentially deal with multiple client prejudices, while remaining responsive to group and individual needs and goals.

"They think they can say anything"

I thought about my extensive experience with groups for male perpetrators of intimate partner violence, in which they regularly expressed sexist, homophobic, or racist views. I am not aware that I had any similar dramatic incidents like my slip, however, I question whether their prejudices affected me more than I realized. I prefer to think that I was mostly successful at containing my feelings; however, it is possible that there were times when my anger negatively affected my interventions.

For example, I recall a group session in which a man, referring to someone who hit his wife saying that he hit his wife "because she was so bitchy and wouldn't shut up. *They* think they can say anything—they feel so powerful now with police and society on their sides, and their good jobs and their fucking independence…no wonder they get hit." I responded by saying, "It sounded like [you are] holding your wife and all of the women in the world responsible for [your] inability to control of himself." He bitterly responded, "You are just taking *their* side." However, the group members identified with my view and said they often "blamed their wives for everything." A few men said they "felt angry at women." However, the man who first commented looked annoyed and said little for the rest of that group session.

Although my intervention may have helped the group, perhaps I was too quick to confront him, rather than process his anger first. Also, the tone in which I delivered the intervention was less than ideal. I likely came across as angry, rather than curious. In hindsight, I think his rage at women reminded me of the Nazi propensity to "blame everything on the Jews."

I reflected on how clinically challenging it could be to promote diversity. Questions such as how, when, and/or whether social workers should address prejudice is very complicated. It is critical that the social worker assess the complex range of historical, social, cultural, and psychodynamic factors that contribute to the client and or group's prejudice. Also, it is possible that the client is not interested in examining his or her beliefs, has other priorities, and/or lacks the capacity for self-reflection. Yet, if the social worker is flooded by intense affect, triggered by the client's prejudiced attitudes, it may be difficult to respond optimally.

In my opinion, the countertransference complexities around diversity often fail to be adequately addressed in social work in general, and social group work. Hence, as a social work educator, I am especially attentive to helping students address these challenges. The following vignette demonstrates my attempt to get students to explore how their countertransference impacts on their ability to effectively work with diversity.

"You all know what those people are like"

In an introductory group-work class, consisting of predominantly women from a range of sociocultural and racial backgrounds, I asked whether anyone would like to present a challenging situation, in which diversity-related issues arose. A young White woman volunteered an example in which she was conducting a support group for elderly clients in a long-term care facility. The group was composed of mostly women, who were all White and from similar socioeconomic backgrounds. She said that the group typically discussed issues such, as their struggles of adjusting to the loss of their partners, health, or independence, and their difficulties adapting to their new residence.

She described how in a recent group, one of the members felt angry at a nurse who had been rude to her, and the client told the other group members: "You all know what *those* (black) people are like." Then a number of people in the group nodded. The group did not display any outward dissent toward her remark, and they then discussed their dislike of certain staff members, the quality of the food, and concerns about their deteriorating health. The student said that she felt "uncomfortable" with the client's comment and the group's failure to challenge her, but she was not sure how to intervene—so she decided not to say anything. She said she was uncertain about whether she had done "the right thing" and asked the class what they thought.

The majority of the students thought that she should have said something. They suggested, for example, that she should have taken the time to "review or establish group rules around racist comments." Another student volunteered how one of her clients made a sexist remark (in a group for people who were recently separated), and she said she reminded them that, "sexist remarks are unacceptable in this group." Then a student said that she thought that perhaps her classmate did the right thing, as "it probably would not have helped to center her out." The class seemed uncertain about the right intervention but leaned toward the idea that she needed to say something that addressed the client's prejudiced remark.

I said that the students made a lot of interesting suggestions, but they had said little about how they "felt" about the client's remark. My inquiry unleashed a lot of comments and emotion. The student who presented said that she felt "anxious and angry." She said that her client's comments, "reminded [her] of her grandparents, who had racist views," and she found that, "it was a waste of time to try to get them to change their opinion." Another student said that she felt angry and that she "hated to hear prejudice." She added, "As social workers, we are obligated to stop it." Some students gave examples when they were hurt by sexist or racist comments.

"It's hard to think clearly when you are furious"

I then asked the class to consider how and whether their feelings might have affected their (recommended) interventions. One student said, "It is hard to think clearly when you are furious!" I said that now that the class had discussed their feelings, that they might be more able to take a step back and assess various interventions. They agreed. I suggested we might first try to further consider the meaning of the client's prejudiced comment.

One student said, "Since the client's nurse had been rude, perhaps the client was getting back at her." Another student said, "Perhaps that woman was angry about being in a nursing home and she was taking it out on all Black people." A student then said that in "the woman's generation, it was probably OK to be prejudiced, so it was part of her culture." A student then said she thought that sometimes in groups people say inappropriate things to "deflect attention away from other issues."

"Okay, but what do you think she should have done?"

I emphasized that prejudice is driven by a range of cultural, social, and personal factors and suggested that all these elements should be considered in formulating an intervention. Then a student said, "OK, but what do *you* think she should have done?"

Ideally, there would have been time for a group role-play, but we had little time left. I indicated that it is always easier to make suggestions in hindsight, but I offered one alternative: I recommended that instead of, and or in addition to setting group rules about prejudice, they might try to "utilize the group process."

For example, I said that after the client said, "You know what *those* people are like," the worker might have gently called the groups' attention to her remark, and asked the members "how they felt" about her comment. A student said, "Maybe somebody would have said they felt offended, and it could have led to more discussion." I added that perhaps the class's anger reflected what some of the group members felt.

However, I added, it was possible that the group members could have ignored the intervention or supported the prejudiced remark. I emphasized that my focus on trying to get the group members reflect on how they felt might have helped some members begin think about their prejudices. I said that I understood that the worker felt it was important to set limits, however, some group members may have experienced her intervention as a "scolding," thus they may have stopped making prejudiced remarks, but withheld their beliefs.

I said that perhaps there was no absolute right or wrong answer. The important thing was to carefully consider our interventions and evaluate whether the intervention helped. We discussed the importance of timing and tact.

With respect to timing, a student shared her work with a homeless client who had homophobic beliefs. He was also struggling with addiction and suicidal thoughts. She felt she could not address this issue when he was in crisis and was uncertain if she could ever address it with him. However, the student expressed her concern that we might be tacitly condoning prejudiced beliefs if we say nothing. I stressed the importance of "good clinical judgment, and considering the client's best interests."

I ended the class by disclosing the story about my client who expressed anti-Semitic views. A student said, "After all your experience that happened to you!" I thought that the class was relieved, as perhaps they felt that we were all in the same boat!

I learned a great deal from my mistake, the men's groups, and group-work class. Even with insight, and advanced training, we all make errors, especially around charged issues such as prejudice. Thus, a critical element for diversity-competent practice is our openness to ongoing self-reflection.

SEARCHING FOR MEANING AND MORE

"It is not freedom from conditions, but it is freedom to take a stand toward the conditions."

Viktor E. Frankl

Insiders in an Empty World

Maria A. Gurrola

We are insiders and outsiders depending on the setting, activity, or function. As we move through different stages in our lives our identity changes and adapts depending on the situation.

As a girl growing up in Mexico with ten brothers and sisters I learned to speak up and be competitive. Participating in an economy in which women are the main caretakers and responsible for the new generation, there was little opportunity to contribute to the workforce. Priority was given to men as breadwinners and providers.

My opportunities changed when I moved to the United States as a young adult, yet even when women have more opportunities, we earn less than men. Furthermore, now I am expected to participate in the workforce and be a caregiver for the next generation. Although this is changing in the United States, women continue to be responsible for children's upbringing and well-being.

Multiple identities

Gender is part of my identity, but I have more than one identity that can limit or advance my opportunities for success. This became clear to me when I moved to the United States.

For example, language was one of the dimensions of my identity that was a barrier to my becoming an insider. Everywhere I went I was an outsider. As long as I pretended I understood what was going on and I was not asked a question it worked, it was great. I remember a White woman telling me that as long as I did not speak I could pass as White.

As the years went by I learned English. Now, I understand what others say and I can speak. Nonetheless, I am still not an insider because of my accent, and my English is not perfect or as good as some would like.

I also learned that even before I speak or before others physically see me, my name is also part of my identity. My name is part of my introduction to others. It may lead them to make assumptions about who I am and where I come from. It can be used to categorize me an insider or outsider.

My journey to and through academia

As social workers, because of the nature of our profession, we often work with diverse groups. Academia provides a great opportunity to teach and provide knowledge to our students. Academia requires educators to work in groups, to create the best curricula for preparing future social workers. In academia there are also administrators and personnel working to structure the environment and provide resources for educators to best engage their students.

University professors can be part of the teaching faculty, administration, or both. Although traditional social work principles are grounded in values of inclusion and social justice, having someone different in one of these groups can create conflict. Difference in the group may be represented by gender, gender identity, race, color, age, country of origin, education, language, and other variables.

In my journey to and through academia it has been an ongoing struggle for me in finding the right fit. Acceptance in a faculty or administrative group does not only happen with people inside the small group but also by people outside the group. For example, besides being accepted to the "inner" group in the school, others still see me as a student in the university. I am often asked about my status in the university until the word *faculty* is seen atop my identification card or associate professor on my business card. This also happens outside the university.

In the local or professional community I am quite often not considered to be a professor. Often, it is required for me to present my business card for me to be considered an insider by people outside the small group. After people see my card, some will comment, "great job" or "this is impressive" or "what a great accomplishment."

When I decided to continue my education after earning my masters in social work, I was working in direct practice providing behavioral health services to adolescents. It was frustrating for me to see families receiving limited services, no medication when the needed it, and long waiting periods to receive case management or counseling services. I wanted to do something to provide better and more appropriate services, culturally and linguistically, for families with a lack of insurance and particularly undocumented immigrants. I decided to advance my education.

The PhD program

As I began taking classes in the PhD program, I learned about social work policy and history, among many other subjects. One class was about how to teach, so I understood that probably I would be doing some teaching. I also took statistics and research methodology, as I would be expected to do some research too.

As I went through the program I talked to different people including research faculty, teaching faculty, and others. I learned the basics about how to look for a job and create a CV (Curriculum Vitae). I learned about the importance of tenure-track position and publishing to be able to get tenure. Looking back, I was on information overload. It was difficult for me to absorb that besides preparing for a tenure-track position I needed to relocate.

I do not remember learning about the structure, politics, or administration in a university. Maybe I needed to learn that on my own, I thought. In my previous involvement in a university I would simply go to class and go back to work or home. Therefore, my transition to becoming an insider in one of these groups was not easy. It was complicated understanding the different layers of structure and power within a department.

My first tenure-track position

As an immigrant, a woman, a Latina, a mother, and a first-generation college graduate I had no background information regarding the roles and structure within academia. I learned a great deal during my first tenure-track position. First, I concentrated on learning about the tenure process and how I could succeed and obtain tenure. I knew there was a chairperson of the program and others who were in charge of different programs. I worked in a teaching university and preparing to teach and learning about tenure took 100% plus of my time. Later, I learned that junior faculty members were protected from administration for them to concentrate on their tenure package. Yet I wondered, did protection mean isolation and lack of information or transparency?

I was a faculty member in a school where many considered me an insider. But I felt that some were not as welcoming as others, not accepting me as one of them. As I continued learning about the tenure process, I also learned about the power and influence of tenured faculty as well as the members of the tenure and promotion committee. As an earning-tenure-track faculty member I remembered what I learned in school and how important it was to follow the guidelines for promotion and tenure.

After my 2nd-year evaluation I also learned that besides following the guidelines for promotion and tenure I needed to be aware of who was in the tenure and promotion committee, their background and their views regarding the school and the university's mission. This was not taught in any of my classes, and I was not advised of this by any of my faculty colleagues inside or outside the school and/or university. I learned how to maneuver my package to fit the university, college, and school and to satisfy the tenure and promotion committee members. I believe this is the first time I realized how a small part of administration works and that I needed to pay attention to who I am working with regardless if I was in an administrative role or not.

It seemed that there were two groups in a school: faculty and administration. I considered myself an insider in the faculty group, even when I knew that everyone in the school did not see me as an insider.

My learning continued as much as my curiosity. I asked an administrator how she got to her position. She confided that it was through a favor.

As I got closer to tenure I was asked to be a program coordinator. I remembered what I was told regarding administration. I was not interested in becoming an administrator except there was the need within the school to participate in this role.

As I began learning about this role I more clearly started to see the lines between the two groups: faculty and administration. I became aware of the differences and similarities as well as the connection between the two groups. I also realized that it can be difficult to be an insider in both groups at the same time, because as you become involved in one you have to reduce your time and energy in the other.

Group dynamics are also different when participating in two groups at the same time. Faculty members might not trust you because you also participate in the administration group. Participating in the two groups does not mean that you are accepted as an insider in either one.

I have been learning about how to manage these two roles together as faculty and administrator.

I enjoyed being in the faculty group because I like the connection with the students. After some time in administration I also see the importance of being a part of securing and maintaining resources for the betterment of the school.

Socializing first-generation students

The social work profession has many avenues of practice. Being in academia has provided me with the opportunity to be in front of a new generation of social workers who are going out into the world to provide services. I have used my experiences and the different dimensions of my identity to create teaching moments in class.

First-generation and minority students begin their education at a different level. If they are able to complete their education, they need the assistance of mentors to be able to acclimate to their work setting.

Often minority professionals do not have mentors who can lead them in the right direction. As minority professionals participate in professions where they are outnumbered, they may be treated as outsiders. Throughout my education, since I arrived in this country, I have met many people who have been very helpful. At the same time I met others who took advantage of me because I did not know how everything worked.

Social justice is a key tenet of social work, yet it cannot be taken for granted. It remains a challenge. Native Americans, African Americans, and Latinos have the highest dropout rate and have the highest rates of incarceration in this country. There is a lack of adequate social services for minority groups and the services that exist are not culturally or linguistically appropriate.

Education, formal and informal, can be used for minorities to advance. As social workers, regardless of the setting in which we practice we need to create environments of inclusion. We need to welcome and mentor outsiders, allowing them to learn the steps for success, instead of closing the doors and excluding them because they are different. Social workers in academia can use their access to students to teach a culture of inclusion where everyone belongs regardless of their identity or where they come from.

The new generation of social workers has a different perspective of who we are as a nation. We have students that have struggled growing up and have been touched by a social worker. I believe that these students will promote a culture of inclusion.

Reflecting back, moving forward

As I reflect on my experience navigating academia, I wonder if there was a reason why I did not learn about administration earlier in my career. Is there a reason to keep administration and faculty groups separate? Why did it take me several years to learn about the politics of tenure and promotion? Was it just my experience? I learned from some colleagues that it is beneficial to actively participate in both, yet others talked about the two groups as if they are separate and disconnected from each other.

As I continue thinking about my position in academia I go back to my experience as a social work practitioner in an agency. Many supervisors and administrators did not see clients. They were making sure that we were able to do our job and that our community received the services they needed. As individuals each of us fit into roles in which we function best. We need to use these roles to create change in our communities.

We have a long way to go as a nation to embrace diversity. As social workers we continue the mission of social justice, embracing difference and advancing equal opportunity, and creating genuine encounters that support acceptance and inclusion. Those of us who choose to be social work educators share the responsibility for engaging and socializing a new generation of social workers to step out and change the world.

Women Faculty of Color in a Predominantly White Institution: A Natural Support Group

Edna W. Comer, Catherine K. Medina, Lirio K. Negroni, and Rebecca L. Thomas

As women faculty of color in a Predominantly White Institution (PWI) we face a myriad of obstacles including marginalization, isolation, and the constant struggle to find balance between our personal and professional identities. Although we are privileged to be working in higher education, we are baffled by the inequalities we must endure to survive and be successful. Yet we have found ways to address our realties, let our voices be heard, and work to affect positive change for those who will follow us in academia. Our story is about how we created a circle of support through a natural support group that helped us to better understand, cope and function in the academe.

Marginalization

Our experiences with marginalization mirror what we have learned from the literature, research, and other women faculty of color in PWIs across the United States. The dominant culture in academia advances meritocracy, encourages free expression and the search for truth, and prizes the creation of neutral and objective knowledge for the betterment of society (Gonzalez & Harris, 2012). Yet these values do not fully reflect the multidimensional aspects of our lives. In a diverse society there are many subjective truths, ways of knowing, and types of knowledge that are contradictory to academia's dominant culture. For example, a neutral and objective knowledge perspective can deny the intersectionality of oppressive constructs that influence our human agency and everyday existence. We, as women faculty of color, frequently find ourselves presumed to be incompetent scholars, teachers, and participants in academic governance. According to the Asian-East Indian member of our group, "It is not uncommon that my ideas or inquires raised in public spaces are often attributed to others. A good idea or an informative fact becomes someone else's. I become highly invisible."

As the African American member of our group remembers, "A White male colleague attempted to encourage me during the tenure process by assuring me that 'people of color are always granted tenure.'" We are aware that hiring women of color in PWIs is often perceived as advantageous because of their gender and race rather than their capabilities as scholars. We know that this perpetuates a subtle message of inferiority and incompetence. A Latina member of our group recalled of a similar incident from the time she was a doctoral student:

> I passed my qualifying exams and was told by a peer that I had passed because I was a person of color. Similarly, at my dissertation defense a peer attributed my achievement to the institution's generous act of passing me as a way to help me as a person of color.

Each one of us has a story to tell about being marginalized by racism in the form of microaggressions such as erroneous comments by colleagues about our professional qualifications and the quality and subject matter of our research. Because each of us often studies issues affecting communities of color, we often hear that unless our groups are compared with the White counterpart they have no meaning. When are studies of communities of color relevant for discourse without the White counterpart?

At the same time that women faculty of color are expected to be the face of diversity for their programs and to prove themselves with their colleagues, students often challenge their professors of color. In preparing this narrative we read about the response of a student to an assistant professor and native of Ghana (Marbley, Wong, Pratt, & Jaddo, 2011). When given a grade for her classroom performance the student responded, "What gives you the right to judge" (p. 168).

Isolation

As women faculty of color we experience physical and intellectual isolation. We are under-represented in academia and especially in PWIs—sometimes being the only one, or one of only a few in our school or department, which helps to explain our feeling isolated and invisible. For example, one of the Latina members of our group has written about the underrepresentation of Latina faculty. This under-representation often silences the discourse on diversity with White mainstream students as well as other students of color. She explains:

> I feel guilty if I talk positively about Puerto Ricans because the students can only associate poverty and immigration issues with this group. They often fail to see this group's bicultural richness and resiliency against all odds. I find it necessary to state in all my classes that I am Latina.

As our natural support group coalesced, all four of us felt that having a connection with a person of color, or a woman faculty from one's race or ethnic group, was an important source of strength and encouragement to help us to persevere in a stressful and competitive academic setting.

We experienced intellectual isolation brought on by behaviors and attitudes that dismissed our efforts and suggested that our work and contributions were insignificant. One reason for our isolation is the lack of opportunity for collaboration on various scholarly initiatives with other faculty. One of our Latina group members provides an example of the time that her social work program was organizing a committee to discuss strategies for recruitment of people of color into the doctoral program:

> I was not asked to be a member in spite of my expressed desire to join the committee. My research endeavors and expertise in the area of recruitment and retention of Latinas into social work education are well known. I was an active member when our national organization had the first task force on the recruitment of Latin@ social workers. My knowledge and experiences were ignored.

The other Latina member of our support group remembers being a part of a peer group intended to discuss and obtain feedback on faculty's research projects:

> On one occasion a White colleague presented her research on working with children of color who were being singled out and suspended for aggressive behaviors. I inquired about her strategies for entering into and engaging the study group and the parents. I did so because in my research experience working with diverse racial and ethnic groups has always been challenging in terms of outreach, engagement and trusting the research goals. I wondered about my colleague's strategies. My colleague did not welcome my inquiry and responded that she had conferred with a person of color who did not have these concerns.

As faculty, we often are newcomers to a world defined and controlled by discourses that do not address our realities, affirm our intellectual leadership and contributions, or seriously examine the multidimensionality of being women of color in a White institution. We have experienced being located on the periphery rather than in the mainstream of teaching and research. Often, we are expected to focus our teaching and research on our specific demographic group. Yet the pursuit of that pathway has resulted in our work being minimized. Sometimes it is seen as anti-intellectual and of little benefit in the mainstream of the academy, especially if we have a different perspective in our teaching, research or publication record.

Professional identity

How faculty of color see their role may differ from the expectations of the academy. Our individuality as women of color is based on values of collectivity, reciprocity, relationality, and connectivity. In contrast, in our experience and conversations with colleagues, we found that PWIs reward individual effort, competition, and commitment to the institution's bureau-cratic guidelines. We often face the dilemma of how to adhere to our individual and cultural values while doing what it takes to "win a battle" in the academy. One of our support group members provides an example:

> As a faculty member in the Puerto Rican Latino Studies Project I am identified with Latina issues and for mentoring Latina students. I often feel a sense of responsibility for the success of students of color. I agree with the sentiments of Carmen González as cited in Turner (2002), that Latina faculty frequently perceive their educational attainment as a way to better prepare themselves to give back to their communities, and increase opportunities for all. There is the recognition that several generations before you have paved the road for your success.

Still another one of our support group recalls being given advice by a colleague to give less time to the community and the Puerto Rican Studies Project:

> She said to me that the reciprocity and connectivity that I felt in my community would likely interfere with my efforts toward tenure and promotion. I wanted to be tenured, but not at the expense of my commitment as a Latina social worker to the community initiatives that impacted youth and addressed violations of human rights. I decided to work extra hard in order to meet institutional expectations without abandoning my other commitments and priorities.

We have read about and talked with one another about a concept called "working identity." This concept suggests that women and people of color may sometimes alter their identities to prevent discrimination and stereotyping in the workplace. We concede that we have spent considerable time and creative energy countering situations that arise because of the conflict between the values we hold for ourselves and the expectations others have of us. However, we remain steadfast in our willingness to illuminate our personal identities, claim our voice and power, and create and advance discourse that addresses our realities and affirms our intellectual contributions.

Our natural support group

Toni Morrison (1970) wrote, "There is nothing more to say—except why? But since why is difficult to handle, one must take refuge in how" (p. 9). We agree with Morrison, that the better question to address about the challenges of being in the academe at this time is not why, but how to cope in an institutional climate in which we are often presumed to be incompetent.

We are African American, Puerto Rican (two of us) and Asian-East Indian. We are tenured associate faculty at a Research One University. We achieved tenure and promotion during the expected time period. The num-ber of years we have been at the university ranges from 9 to 17 years. Each of us arrived at the University at different times. Two of us arrived within a year of each other and the other two 5 and 6 years later, respectively. None of us knew each other prior to beginning work at the university. Our relationships and support group evolved naturally, by being in the same place and feeling marginalized and isolated. We shared a feeling that our sense of professional identity was at stake. Often, we referred to these feelings, as "losing our spirit."

Coming together as a group helped us to cope with our positions as faculty of color in a PWI. Our natural support group helped us manage the stress related to our roles. The group validated our individual and collective professional value and worth, counteracted our isolation, and helped us to build and nurture our friendships.

We have no designated time to get together. Yet we always make the time—an impromptu meeting in the corridor to check-in with each other, a brief closed door office meeting to offer encouragement and support, a space for us to express feeling overwhelmed or needing affirmation. Here is an example of how our Asian-East Indian colleague describes getting together with the group:

> I developed a ritual that upon arrival in the building I walk down to the offices of my colleagues to greet them and check in. It is often a quick hello, to share a story, or sit awhile. I want to let them know I am in my office and available to support them if they need me.

We did not immediately connect with each other and do not recall the specifics of how we joined together as a group. We think that the close proximity of our offices was one factor. Interestingly our offices were all on the same floor and hallway. It was fortunate that all our offices are located in the same corridor.

Another reason for forming our support group was that we shared the relocation experience of transitioning to a new job in a new state, with no friends or personal acquaintances. We became family to each other—a chosen family. On a personal level we take care of each other in different ways, we advise each other and we do fun things together. For example, as RT observes:

> I sought out their opinions, experiences, advice and expertise in multiple ways. It was not a systematically planned effort but rather a natural affinity space among the group for levity, humor, encouragement, clarification and just an everyday checking. The group did not evolve because of a particular incident but as we began to create social capital amongst ourselves we moved from bridging to bonding. We participate in social activities together—my home often became the gathering space to break bread, listen to music, celebrate our cultures, try new things, develop ideas and get feedback. We plan social activities as desired and needed. We celebrate each other's accomplishments and good days.

CM notes, "Different factors converged to bring us together as a group but I think the key factor has been our support for each other during preparation for tenure and promotion." EC adds that "LN and I were going through the tenure process at the same time. We worked together and kept each other informed about procedures."

CM continues:

> The collective spirit of the group was instrumental as I navigated the tenure process. There was an unspoken but known feeling that each of us wanted the other to succeed as a scholar. The unspoken but felt need was that each of us believed in the potential of the other.

LN adds:

> We all agreed that the tenure and promotion process was a major strand that unified us. However, our professional commitment to advancing knowledge and providing mentorship to others is crucial.

In a naturally formed group, members needs and desires signify its purpose. Our group provides emotional support and social connection and helps us to adapt to and manage our roles as women faculty of color in a PWI. According to LR:

> The group has provided me with validation, opportunities for reflection, self-affirmation, and clarity as to the external and internal institutional and faculty forces, celebration of accomplishments, nurturing and help with family and personal matters.

RT observes:

> The group is a sounding board for some of my scholarship ideas and research. It is a place I debrief after teaching a class that went well or horribly wrong. A place to share personal stories, celebrate birthdays, holidays and major achievements. It is a place in which I can find comfort when I encounter difficult life crossroad.

CM remarks:

> The support of the group nurtures and helps us to understand our struggles and accept our successes. It helps us as women of color to manage the challenges associated with scholarship and excellence in PWI and how to use our strength to overcome and thrive in the academe.

EC adds, "The group provides a safe and nurturing environment. It allows for reality testing that illuminates both my strengths and challenges."

In naturally formed groups it is uncommon to have consciously planned interventions, but rather activities that occur as needed and are helpful to members in achieving their goals. We have engaged in a number of activities —discussions related to professional achievements and social events to celebrate personal and life transitions. EC explains, "We attend birthday and holiday celebrations and events to support each other receiving recognition such as community awards or acknowledgement." LN goes on to stress the importance of our being there for one another beyond the context of the academy, "We accompany each other to medical appointments and medical emergencies and other personal crisis that require support." EC adds, "We make time to discuss daily work and personal life situations, and current and world events. All of us agree that, simply stated, we check in on each other."

Natural support groups do not have planned endings or terminations. They continue as long as there is an interest and need and as long as members are willing to invest the time. We have not considered the group ending or thought about where it is headed; rather, we focus on the moment. LN wonders:

Is this going to remain a friendship group? As we move toward retirement or relocate what will happen to the group? We will no longer need support around our work and lives as social work educators. Over time we may need to redefine our purpose and focus.

RT says:

The group has become my friend. I am able to express and be myself honestly. I know that I will be understood through my multiple identities and, as tough questions are asked, have the confidence that the group will be patient with me as I find words to express thoughts, feelings and ideas. As each of us transitions toward our individual goals, our supportive allies in the group become a sounding board.

CM emphasizes the group's value in terms of personal and professional growth:

Because we are tenured faculty we have the responsibility to navigate academia with a sense of power and human agency, and to be open to discovery and to contributing to advancing social work. As a group, we continue to be solidified in giving voice to different perspectives in teaching, research and publication in countering dominant ideologies or eliminating subordination in the academy.

EC observes, "I really have not thought about life without the group."

We hope that by sharing our story it will help others to see the benefits in joining together to be part of a natural support group, especially in competitive settings that result in marginalization, isolation and questioning one's professional identity. Reflecting here on our experiences of "friends supporting friends" has been awesome.

The proximity of our offices, the mutual need to form social and professional bonds and our growing ability to relate supportively to one another around the tenure and promotion process were some of the factors that drew us together. The respect we have for one another, the willingness to support and be supported by one another, pre- and posttenure, and the good times and laughter we have being together will likely keep our group going for a long time.

References

González, C. G., & Harris, A. P. (2012). The "liberal" ivory tower often discriminates against women of color. In G. Guitierrez, Y. F. Niemann, C. G. Gonzalez, & A. P. Harris (Eds.), *Presumed incompetence: The intersections of race and class for women in academia* (pp. 1–14). Boulder, Colorado: University of Colorado Press.

Marbley, A., Wong, A., Pratt, C., & Jaddo, L. (2011). Women faculty of color: Voices, gender, and the expression of our multiple identities within academia. *Advancing Women in Leadership, 31,* 166–174.

Morrison, T. (1970). *The bluest eye.* New York, NY: Washington Square Press.

Turner, C. S. V. (2011). Women of color in academe: Living with multiple marginality. *The Journal of Higher Education, 73*(1), 74–93.

Healing Through Group Work

Bharati Sethi

On a crisp September morning on my way to facilitate the first Peace and Diversity advisory group meeting, I stopped for a few moments at a park a block away from the community center where the group meeting was being held. The trees were clothed with vibrant gold, purple, yellow, green, and red leaves. I watched the squirrels in childlike wonder. They were busy searching for nuts hidden under the fallen leaves. As I walked through the pathway dodging the walnuts falling from the trees, the wind gently stroked my hair. I liked the rustling sound of the leaves beneath my feet. Stepping out of the park I glanced behind me one more time. After residing in Canada for 15 years, the autumn grandeur still took my breath away.

Without warning, dark clouds hovered over the sky outside the community center. I held tightly to the silk dupatta around my neck—a gift from my friend Vanaja that had survived the long journey from India to Canada. It made me feel closer to her and less anxious. She was my rock all through the childhood years in India. Perhaps it was the "role model" image, I thought, that was making me unusually nervous. Several local media articles and interviews had recently portrayed me as a "success story"; after all, I had endured immigration hardships, washed dishes, cleaned houses, and worked in factories to support my dream of achieving a PhD. No!! It wasn't the role model image that had stopped me at the doorstep of the community hall, one hand on the door handle. Through the glass door I stared at the sign at the entrance, "Have you been a victim of racism and/or hate crime? Join the Peace and Diversity group." Without warning, flashbacks enveloped me.

I was barely age 22 years. I was walking home after my evening shift at a restaurant. That cold winter night I narrowly escaped the attack of three White men chasing me and jeering, "Paki, go back to your country." I wasn't even from Pakistan. I was from India. It was clear to me that this act was motivated by hate, and I was being intimidated and targeted due to the intersection of my race, ethnicity, perhaps gender, and immigration status. As per the Criminal Code of Canada (Minister of Justice, 2014), hate crime is an offense. Section 319 of the Criminal Code of Canada states:

Everyone who, by communicating statements in any public place, incites hatred against any identifiable group where such incitement is likely to lead to a breach of the peace is guilty of (a) an indictable offence and is liable to imprisonment for a term not exceeding 2 years; or (b) an offence punishable on summary conviction. (Minster of Justice, 2014, p. 353)

I did not report the attack to the police as I was then working on a foreign work permit and I did not want to be sent back to India. Taking a deep breath, I brought myself back to the present. It was now clear to me why I had agreed to join the Peace and Diversity group.

I was pleasantly greeted at the reception desk by a Muslim woman in her fifties. After asking the purpose of my visit she led me to a small comfortable and well-lit room. The sight of multicolored fall leaves through the glass window calmed my nerves. I waited for the other members to arrive. I had introduced myself, as the chair of the advisory group, to the seven individuals through e-mail but this was the first time we were going to meet face to face. Our project, I felt, was very important. As members of the community Peace and Diversity advisory group, we were entrusted the challenging task of finding innovative ways to reduce "hate crimes" in this community. Over the past few years, there had been a rise in hate crimes in this middle-sized urban-rural region in southern Ontario with a population of approximately 237,339. This region was traditionally not an immigrant reception zone for immigrants of color, but in recent years had experienced migration from non-European nations. It was also evident from the unlawful hate-motivated incidents that some members of the community were not open to people of diverse sexual orientation. As a community-based researcher, an advocate, and an academic, I lived for such moments.

One by one, other members joined me. I noticed that the attendees were of Asiatic, Middle Eastern, African, and European origin. All of us were immigrants. During the introductions, I heard brief accounts of their lives pre- and postmigration. As a one-year pilot project, we were granted limited finances for activities that would reduce hate crimes in this community toward vulnerable groups. We only had a year to make some positive changes. There was no time to waste. Immediately after introductions, we began a brainstorming session. I was taken aback by the chaos and hostility in the room. We barely tolerated each other. An intense argument emerged about "which group is the most oppressed" (i.e. people of diverse sexual orientation, immigrant women, Muslims, or Asians, etc.). Observing carefully, I wondered if members had brought their "unattended pain" with them and if indeed their wounded self was interfering from focusing on the task at hand. For instance, a gay European male member of the group felt that our efforts should be targeted at the gay community. A female Muslim member was very vocal about the oppression of Muslims in society post-911and wanted the group to focus on the oppression of Muslim women. As the chair I had to remain unbiased, yet, I was still disturbed by the "Paki, go home" sounds that disturbed the stillness of that night not so long ago and have continued to haunt me since.

The next day, after a sleepless night, I e-mailed the members suggesting that during our next meeting I would like us to share our experiences of racism and hate. I encouraged each member to do so over a potluck dinner. Late into the night we listened to our individual and collective stories. There were narratives of oppression, resilience, successes, suffering, and celebration. Ethnicity, gender, immigration status, sexual identity, and geography (living in an urban or rural region) intersected in these accounts to shape our experiences. Lost in their stories, I barely heard a group member call out my name. Her voice seemed to echo from somewhere far away. Brushing the uninvited tears from my eyes, I stood up. Overflowing with awe from the testimonies I had just heard, I addressed the group members, "Hello, my name is Bharati. Like you, I am a survivor of hate crimes." It was clear that each member had a painful and frightening brush with hate. Joining the Peace and Diversity group and taking an active stand to reduce hate crime in our community, we perhaps secretly hoped, would bring us some healing. Perhaps, we could take back our power from the perpetrators.

During our third meeting, there was new energy in the room. It seemed to me that by making ourselves vulnerable enough to share the skeletons in our closet with others, we were feeling lighter. At least I was. No! This was not a support group for victims of hate crimes, but I learnt that we cannot individually and/or collectively affect change unless we tackle the skeletons in our closets. Moving forward, there was a consensus that we were not going to play the "oppression game" of who was more oppressed, rather, target our activities at reducing hate crimes. Our individual and collective goal was to be a catalyst in promoting peace, eliminating discrimination, and establishing an inclusive culture in the community where people of different races and sexual orientation can live in peace and harmony. That is the task we were entrusted with regardless of our individual social locations and experiences. We would do that through education, community forums, and art. Hate against Muslims, women, gays, lesbians, and so on was hate, and regardless of which social category we identified with (in regards to our gender, race, class, ability, orientation, etc.) we were familiar with the pain of hate. It pierced deep into our soul. Over the next few meetings I recognized that to do empowering group work and bring about positive change, first, it is important to be clear about the intentions and motivations of joining a particular group. Second, I needed to make those intentions transparent to those with whom I was going to work closely for the next year. After all, most of us volunteer for projects for which we have passion.

As a chairperson of the advisory group, I found myself wearing several hats—facilitator, mediator, counsellor, leader, and so on. I was the captain guiding the ship. Even though the task was demanding, having established "trust" with the group through making my intentions, motivations, goals, and pain transparent, made the job much easier. We were bonded by our individual and collective stories. Without peace in my heart and peace within the group with whom I was going to work on a very personal issue I could not bring peace in the community. I also understood that just because I had bared the skeleton from my closet to the group, the issue wasn't necessarily resolved. For instance, each time I would read about rape, attacks on Muslims, or a gay store that was burnt down, I could feel the pain and fear of hate crimes all over again. As a chairperson it was my role to ensure that I did not lose members to exhaustion and lack of motivation. I introduced reflection and debriefing sessions at the end of every meeting. Individually and collectively we reflected on recent hate crime incidents in the community and how they affected us. The feedback I received was that members found these sessions vital to staying motivated and strong. These sessions also strengthened the bond between us. We were much stronger as a group than individually. We encouraged and supported each other. It is also important to recognize the value of humor in group work and in working with painful issues. We laughed out loud. We laughed heartily. We laughed often. Until this experience, I had never imagined that group work could be so healing. Because we were so transparent with each other, our work in the community was very effective. We organized panel presentations, distributed flyers, brought people of different faiths together to voice their views about hate crimes, and even proposed a gay pride day. Whenever a conflict emerged we solved it with faith that each member's input was equally valuable. By year end we had utilized the finances entrusted to us to promote peace and diversity. Even though there was still a lot of work to be done, I would like to believe that our efforts made the community more inclusive. We did that together. From barely tolerating each other in the first meeting, we embraced mutual empathy and celebrated the dimensions of diversity within our group. We did that through genuine encounter and embodied actions. At the concluding meeting when I embraced every group member I was no longer feeling disembodied as I had felt in the first meeting.

Having been a member of many different groups, I recognize that not all the groups will offer opportunities for healing, but if we treat every encounter as sacred, it can be empowering. Instead of the need to be right, if we can just for a moment put our ideologies aside and respect diverse epistemologies, we can learn from the other group members. It is important to keep in mind that Canada is a multicultural country. Diversity is our nation's identity. The following group norms helped me navigate various groups regardless of my interest and expertise and group demographics, mission, and complexity with mutual empathy. I explain them under the Acronym DIVERSITY

> D—Delving deep into issues
> I—Showing Interest in other members' views
> V—Applauding other members' Victories
> E— Encouraging members to participate
> R—Having Respect for other group members
> S—Sharing humor
> I—Communicate from "We" rather than "I" position
> T—Being Tolerant of diverse opinions
> Y—Being very clear about WHY I joined the group and WHY I continue
> to stay.

In conclusion, I would like to add that empathetic encounter is possible when we are vigilant of not just our oppression but our privilege (in terms of age, class, gender, ethnicity, ability, etc.) and recognize that those we meet also dwell at the intersection of privilege and encounter with varying intensity.

Reference

Minister of Justice. (2014). *Criminal code.* Retrieved from http://laws-lois.justice.gc.ca/PDF/C-46.pdf

"Being Accepted" and *"Being Accepted"?*

Jan Fook

I am by official nationality Australian but born of Chinese heritage. Most of the time I call myself "later generation Australian-born Chinese," though this is changing. I left Australia nearly 10 years ago, and I now live in the United Kingdom. I am also of lower middle-class background but happen to have spent more than three decades working in academia, and in the last two decades, as a senior academic. The reason I am telling you this is so that you will get a sense of my complex mix of identities that I am still forging. Being socially different, and creating a meaningful place for me professionally and personally, has been an ongoing task that will continue until the day I die. In this experience I will tell the story of when I came to one particular realization about my own difference. It was a breakthrough moment in understanding my own feelings about social acceptance, in the context of other people's understandings.

Setting the stage

The scene is this: I am leading a small group in a workshop on critical reflection for a group of team leaders in children's services in a London borough. I often conduct these workshops to give people a practical experience of critical reflection, and to help them learn a structured but fluid process for reflecting. In a nutshell, the process involves helping people learn from their own experience by reflecting on a piece of experience (an incident) that is important to them and that they would like to learn from. After an introduction to the theory of critical reflection and the process, I normally begin the practical part of the workshop by using an example of my own incident and asking them to help me undertake some reflection on it. I find that this models the process, but even more importantly, establishes an egalitarian culture and one where it feels more acceptable to risk vulnerability in order to learn. These, to me, are vital components of being open to learning from a critical reflection process, which may unearth unpredictable and sometimes threatening realisations and emotions.

Modelling

I am modelling the critical reflection process by presenting an example of my own experience. The group will help me reflect the specific experience by asking me questions, and undertake dialogue with me, so that I can discover something more about the deeper assumptions which underlie my own thinking and behavior. The session starts in the usual way. I tell them (about eight people, a mix of women and men, a mix of several different ethnicities, and a mix of ages) about a small incident that for me is significant to my learning. It happens a lot, I find it frustrating, and would like to try and understand more about what it means, so that I can change how I see it and how I might act in the future. Simple enough. The incident I tell is, at face value, very ordinary:

> I am in a new position, with a new university. I am in an all-day meeting which involves some quite senior people in my university. The meeting is to plan the next year's strategic activities. Partway through the meeting I begin to realize that I don't think I understand what is happening. We do not seem to be following the agenda, people do not seem to be responding to what others have said, I cannot tell what (if any) decisions are being made, and slowly I become more silent, not wishing to speak up in case I expose my ignorance. I leave the meeting frustrated and annoyed, feeling that I have wasted my time and that my voice was not heard.

I tell the story succinctly and with some aplomb. I have presented it many times to many different groups, as part of the numerous critical reflection sessions I have provided. I feel pretty self-assured. But at the same time I believe I am happy to be open to new ideas, to questions that might shake my preconceived reflections, and I am conscious of trying to give this message, so that people will be encouraged to experiment with critical reflection, by experimenting on me, no less. At the same time I am aware that at heart I am pretty certain nothing the group can say will faze me. I feel in control, not necessarily vulnerable as the process suggests one needs to be, in order to be truly open to what might arise.

People start asking me questions. They are trying to help me discover what some of my deeper assumptions might be, as implied by the story of my experience. At the start, the questions are fairly predictable. There is a little apprehension, as people still seem a bit unsure of what they are supposed to be doing, but in general, there is not much tension in the air, as there sometimes is at the start of a new group, when people are unfamiliar with each other and no one wants to break the ice. I am happy about this because I have done my best (I think) to lighten the atmosphere and create a climate of collegiality, so that people will feel comfortable to participate, and to risk losing a little "face" by asking questions, whether or not they are sure they are properly critically reflective.

At first the questions seem fairly "factual", focused on finding out more about the situation......

"Were most meetings run like this?" (Mandy)
"Were you adequately prepared for the meeting?" (Raj)
"Did anyone else speak up about what was happening?" (Aniela)

I don't answer any of these questions directly. Instead I ask why each person has asked what he or she did. In a sense I am asking them to reflect on what was behind their questioning. I wonder (out loud) what it is about my own thinking or assumptions they thought they were trying to help me reflect on.

Their responses are fairly predictable. "I was thinking that you can't have really understood what the meeting was supposed to be about, and that this must have been due to poor preparation," Raj volunteers a bit sheepishly. Everyone laughs, slightly nervous, because the implied judgment may be perceived as a bit harsh, but also because they possibly recognize that this was exactly what they were thinking.

"So was your question about my thinking, or yours Raj?" Poor Raj—I feel a bit sorry to have put him on the spot but the learning moment seems too opportune. He doesn't need to answer this but does grin and nod. "I think I get it," he says.

"So do you want to have a go at asking your question in a different way, which might help me reflect on my thinking about my preparation for the meeting?"

He looks thoughtful and a little pained. I ask the group to try and help him. "How about ... Did you feel adequately prepared for the meeting?'" (Tim) "Better," I said. "You will notice that the way Tim worded that question invited me to focus more on my own thinking (feeling). Perhaps you could also have said, "Do you think you were adequately prepared for the meeting...and if not, what would 'adequate preparation' be for you?"

Nods all round. "Why do you think those questions might help me reflect?" I pause, quickly realizing it might be better to demonstrate a real response and let them work out what it is about the question which helps to elicit reflective responses. "No, better still, I will answer Tim's question for you and you can judge for yourself." I respond with exaggerated thoughtfulness to Tim's question.

"You ask if I felt adequately prepared. Actually, yes, I did think I was adequately prepared. I had the agenda a week beforehand and had been briefed on my role (I had been asked to do a short presentation of ideas for going forward). So for me it was not a matter of preparation at all, *but that my expectations about how a meeting should be run were not met.*" I put significant emphasis on these last words, hoping someone will pick up on the hint regarding my assumptions about how meetings should be run.

"Is that why you think you didn't speak up?" (Julie)

"Because my expectations were not met?" I query.

"Yes, were you feeling there was no place for your voice because you thought the meeting was not being run in the way you wanted"? (Julie)

"Sort of … I think it's more that I was really thrown because the meeting was not run according to my expectations, so I didn't know where I stood." Still reflecting further I go on." It sounds like it must be important to me to know where I stand before I can participate meaningfully … so there's an assumption here about needing to understand before acting I guess." This sounds all a bit wordy and my fear is confirmed when Aniela asks another question which seems to completely disregard the path I am trying to lead the group down.

"Were you the only woman in the room?" (Julie)

Oh no! (I think to myself). Have we learnt nothing about not asking factual questions? Nevertheless I answer…

"No, about half the meeting members were women … but why do you ask?"

"Did you think gender was an element in why you felt you couldn't speak up?" (Julie)

Now that's more like it! "Good question!" I enthuse, and I step out of role slightly to draw out some more learning about the critical reflection process. "It's good to frame it the latter way, because you are trying to get me to think about whether gender is an important issue for me—you are trying to get me to focus on my own assumptions, so framing it this way goes directly to my thinking."

"But everyone wants to be accepted"

There is an almost audible murmur in the room as people try and take in the learning I am outlining here. Back to the process…

> "I would answer this by saying that I don't think I was so aware of my gender but I was certainly aware of other social differences." I look around, almost anticipating their anticipation, wondering what they will make of this. There is silence as they wait for me to continue. It's as if they all think they know what I am going to say, but everyone wants me to say it, not volunteer it themselves.
>
> Clearly I am not of white or of British background. I am Chinese by background, and what's more I am an Australian (in a British context) and I was also, in this instance, new to the job. There were plenty of markers to identify me as different. Being a woman was fairly far down the list.

This is now getting interesting. People are pausing, looking thoughtful. How will they tackle this next issue? I am used to people from more mainstream backgrounds feeling uncomfortable when issues of race raise their heads. They often avoid even using the term, or wait for the racialized person to initiate the conversation.

Julie asks, "These things made you feel different. Do you think you were wanting to feel accepted?" Julie seems to be getting the gist of these questions and is being more direct about getting to the heart of the matter. I have to pause for a while in thinking about this question. I am aware that many in the group are nodding almost imperceptibly, but I am getting a clear message that people feel they have "hit the nail on the head." There is almost a sense of smugness, as if they as a group have gotten "the answer." Perversely this makes me want to not agree, but more than that I detect a small, but nevertheless definite, whir of anger, in my own response.

"No, actually I am not at all worried about being accepted." This sounds a bit stark, and I'm not sure if I can risk being too direct in this setting, so I soften it. "I mean I don't think wanting to be accepted was what was motivating me here."

They are still listening, waiting for me to go on. I can see that they don't seem to understand "not wanting to be accepted," and I'm also starting to feel that they don't believe me. I feel them thinking, "but everyone wants to be accepted" ("especially people who are different") is the latter bit I imagine that I add for myself. I have to choose my words carefully as it dawns on me that perhaps "being accepted" *is* what every mainstream person thinks every marginal person wants! I think this is what this tiny knot of anger is about for me. I might have been completely off the beam here, but it starts a train of thought of private conversation which runs at the back of my head even while I participate outwardly in the group.

Being accepted and *being accepted*

I start to realize that there is "being accepted" and "*being accepted.*" The former implies being accepted in the terms of the group doing the accepting. In other words, it is being accepted as being like the people in the mainstream group. It feels like (to someone from a marginal group) that this is like conferring an honorary "mainstream" status on the marginal person. I have in fact had this kind of thing said to me on many occasions. "Oh, we don't see you as different, because it's your accent we hear, and you sound just like us." (Said to me by Australian students in Australia, in a class on cross-cultural social work when we were discussing our own cultural/ethnic identities). To me this is a form of denying (and perhaps devaluing?) difference, rather than accepting it. This is a similar phenomenon to that noted by Amy Rossiter (1995) when speaking about a women's group in which it was assumed that women of non-White backgrounds were happy to be accorded "equal" status, whether they wanted it! It is another version of White women saying "you're just like us," thinking that a great privilege is being conferred. It is, I guess, a form of positive prejudice that implies that whatever the non-White person is, it must be inferior, to whatever is being conferred by honorary white status.

The other type of "*being accepted,*" which I forcefully realized is what I really wanted, is to be accepted for who and what I thought I was or wanted to be. In this case I think I was saying that I wanted to be accepted as just being me, that is, a person who might happen to have a racialized appearance, and for whom this provided a partial identity, but also someone who was new to the job, comes from another country, but who also had substantial experience, lots of ideas to offer, and for whom admitting confusion about the meeting would not be seen as a sign of incompetence, but an understandable and sensible issue to raise. I felt like being accepted in these terms would be about being accepted in *my* terms.

I struggled to communicate this to the group and found my voice sounding a bit shaky while doing so. This made me realize how important the issue was to me, and as I spoke about it, I had memory flashes of many times in my own life when I had not felt accepted or valued for who or what I thought I was or wanted to be. Incidentally, many of these instances had nothing to do with racial differences but did have a lot to do with being out of kilter socially and ideologically with the mainstream groups in which I found myself at the time. I think I started to realize that the "difference" I felt due to my racialized appearance constituted only a small portion of the concern about nonacceptance I often experience in my personal and professional life. Awareness of my own complex identity of multiple differences made me also aware of the difficulty of feeling accepted for who and what I was. I started to appreciate that it might therefore be very difficult for people, who saw themselves as having more straightforward identities, to appreciate this odd mixture of backgrounds and ideologies which made up who and what I was now.

And yet I didn't really want them to appreciate it all, but just to accept that what I said about myself. I just wanted my own perspective on myself to be heard and accepted as mine. I did not want to be seen as someone striving to be like others, as wanting the same status derived from being socially similar. They did not have to share the same view of me, but they did have to accept that I had a view of myself which might be different from theirs and that this was legitimate. How hard was that?

Deepening my reflection through the group experience

The workshop continued and ended, focusing on how group processes could be used to facilitate reflection. The irony for me was that my own reflection was facilitated in a way that I hadn't anticipated, and that had lasting repercussions for my own sense of self. Being open and true to the process had actually yielded a deeper form of reflection.

Had the group process itself helped me in arriving at this realization about the two forms of acceptance? Yes, I do think that reflecting on my own experience in the context of dialogue with other people actually helped foreground my own perspective in contrast to how I perceived theirs.

Interestingly, this view was reinforced for me when I revisited an auto-ethnographic piece I wrote in which I used a critical self-reflection process to try and understand my own sense of social difference and how I had made meaning of this (Fook, 2014). My learning about social difference and its role in my life takes quite a different tack, not incompatible with the present experience, but goes in quite a different direction and does incorporate the idea of wanting to "fit in" much more than my reflective experience above illustrates. So it is the group experience, and my impression of their collective understanding, which demonstrated to me the more hidden assumptions of other people about acceptance, and how I make myself in that context of other peoples' understandings.

References

Fook, J. (2014). Learning from and researching (my own) experience: A critical reflection on the experience of social difference. In S. Witkin (Ed.), *Narrating social work through Autoethnography* (pp. 120–140). New York, NY: Columbia University Press.

Rossiter, A. (1995). Entering the intersection of identity, form, and knowledge: Reflections on curriculum transformation. *Canadian Journal of Community Mental Health, 14*(1), 5–14. doi:10.7870/cjcmh-1995-0001

Breaking Taboos: The Power of Group Work for First-Generation Scholars

George W. Turner, Michael D. Pelts, and Michelle G. Thompson

Collectively reflecting on the call for papers for this special edition of *Social Work with Groups* served as a reminder for us that groups form in many ways. It also reminded us that what brings people together may be a topical matter and what holds groups together is finding a meaningful bond, a relationship. Our group: Turner (a newly minted PhD faculty), Pelts (a doctoral candidate) and Thompson (a midprogram doctoral student), originally formed to discuss overlapping research interests. We quickly realized that the common bond that connected us was our identities as first-generation scholars (FGS). Over several months, through the regaling of our academic journeys, a collective transformative experience happened. In this narrative, our stories as FGS became the backdrop of our group experience. In the unpacking and reflecting on our group experience, we allowed space for creative work beyond the "real work," avoiding what Malekoff (2001) refers to as "spiritual incarceration" (p. 255). It is here we seek to uncover the value of the social work group experience as a tool for FGS success.

How we met

Our group began to emerge when George, hungry to meet scholars with similar research interests, reached out to Michael after reading an article Michael had published. Even though they lived only 2 hours apart, efforts to meet fell short for months. Persistent, George solidified lunch plans with Michael on the first day of the 2014 Council on Social Work Education (CSWE) Annual Program Meeting in Tampa. Before leaving CSWE, George and Michael realized that not only did their research interests overlap, but also their experiences as FGS. Even in this early stage, George encouraged Michael that these experiences as FGS were ripe for exploring and sharing with others in academia. The two stayed in touch and began to schedule regular meetings via skype to explore their interests.

A few months later at the 2015 Society for Social Work Research (SSWR) Annual Conference in New Orleans, Michael met Michelle during an orientation session for student volunteers. They too quickly bonded over their overlapping research interests and FGS identities.

Within a couple of weeks Michelle was a part of the skype meetings. The three of us started meeting in February 2015, and we continue to meet every couple of weeks. During our meetings, we explore ways to advance our scholarly work and confer about ways to manage the academic terrain. More importantly, we visit. We make time to catch up and check in with one another. This seemingly innocuous ritual is a rich and fundamental process in the weaving together of our collective relationship. Realizing how strongly our backgrounds as FGS influences our experiences in academia, we each took one meeting to share what it was like for us as FGS. We also shared how being a FGS affects us today as we navigate the academy. We captured those narratives, and it is through that lens the social work group principles of mutual aid, inclusion and respect, and breaking taboos (Drumm, 2006) were illuminated.

The FGS experience

George: Mutual aid

As a FGS, I often see glimpses of myself in some of my students: occupying the in-between ...an outsider in your family and within the academy, navigating with trepidation the transition to higher education, and feeling like an imposter. Recalling my own rocky educational path after high school, I was promoted from part time to full-time at Kmart. I remember asking myself, "Is this all there is for me?!" I grew up in a rural, impoverished socioeconomic area and any full-time employment was considered good enough. None of my friends planned on college. Despite being a good student, there was no discussion or expectation to pursue a college degree.

My parents were not only unable to financially support a college education, but also had no point of reference to offer any practical guidance. My mother, a waitress, did not graduate high school and my father was an over-the-road truck driver, who had some college. In fact, they at times were a barrier. Highlighting my "outsider" status was my father's refusal to provide his income information on my financial aid application. My dad's stance that no one had the right to his private information solidified that I was alone on this journey.

Often a source of shame, my status as a FGS was embraced with familiarity and fondness by Michael and Michelle. Our ascribed purpose, research collaboration, gave way to a more pressing interpersonal need: camaraderie, healing, and support. For me, the power within the group process to foster mutual aid was illuminated during our meetings.

I reminisced that leaving for college was embarking on a journey that carried me away from my family, not only geographically, but away from my place in the family. I was abandoning them semester by semester as my formal education and life exposure widened a profound yet unseen gap between them and me. It seemed that my family, straddling between pride and apprehension, saw me as occupying some foreign new space.

Yet I didn't find a replacement family in academia. I was just as much an outsider here too as highlighted when I set out across country for school. Tied to a luggage rack atop my car were black trash bags holding all my clothes. We did not own any luggage. Alone and poorly prepared, my educational journey has often felt risky, uncertain, and like a leap of faith. I've often felt embarrassment in my lack of designer luggage or a decent bon voyage send-off for this adventure of a lifetime. With Michelle and Michael I found camaraderie, a climate of good will in the similarities of our stories. In the building of this group relationship, I have a sense of collegiality. Help is freely given and taken in this work group.

The simple nod of group members seeing all of me was a vulnerable act of healing. Bringing my self-doubt to light has allowed me to unpack this baggage and explore its origins. More importantly it has reaffirmed my place in the academy and highlighted my FGS as a strength to be used in connecting with my students.

In meeting Michelle and Michael I have found a crucial support system. They are not just colleagues to explore scholarly research and writing, but FGS soulmates. They are cheerleaders to encourage my ideas, beacons to illuminate the pathway, and friends to prop me up along my continued adventure through the academy.

Michelle: Inclusion and respect

I recall sitting at a professor's office nearly in tears. I was overwhelmed with the entire PhD program. I told the professor that I am a FGS and did not understand how to navigate academia and all of the unspoken expectations that have been thrust upon me. I stated that some of the students in my program seem to know the right questions to ask or already have the answers. I felt lost, like I did not belong. That professor's response did not make me feel any better. "I'm going to be tough but you need to hear it. Nobody is going to hold your hand. Obtaining your PhD is a very independent process." These statements are replayed over and over. I keep asking for a manual or some type of informal guidance. Apparently there isn't one.

In comparison to George and Michael, my pathway to the PhD program has been quite different and yet in some ways strangely similar. I grew up in a lower middle-class, biracial/bicultural household, in a large Southern sub-urban city. Similar to George and Michael, my father, an African American, was born and raised in a very rural area on a farm in Georgia. However my mother is Caribbean Puerto Rican and spent parts of her life in Puerto Rico and New York.

I was a fairly bright kid during my primary and secondary education. When my parents divorced at age 10, my behavior changed and I often found myself in rough waters at home, in school, and any place where I had the opportunity to act out. Because I was quite bright and despite my outrage and protests, my mother enrolled me into a public college preparatory high school my tenth grade year. Neither my parents nor grandparents graduated from college. They often could not help my siblings and me with our homework. We also knew that they could not afford to send us off to college, however; my family saw the value in obtaining higher education and pushed us to excel academically. Despite my adolescent antics, my mother saw my potential, and I managed to successfully complete my Bachelor's and Master's degree in Psychology before age 26 and enroll in a PhD program that I hope to complete before the age of 40.

I felt a little out of place when I initially shared parts of my upbringing with our group. The various dimensions of difference between us are quite stark. I thought to myself, what in the world would I have in common with middle-aged, White men from rural nowhere? To my surprise, I learned that first-generation status cuts across race, ethnicity, class, and gender. When I share these experiences with George and Michael, they totally get me. They don't tell me to "suck it up" or "get over it." They allow me to vent and also validate my experiences. During our sessions, I know that for that allotted time, my voice will be heard, my feelings will be validated, and I will end the call feeling renewed and energized. They affirm that there is a light at the end of the tunnel. Through the principle of inclusion and respect, George, Michael, and I have found a common ground in our FGS experiences that have proven very valuable to how I reflect upon my own journey moving forward.

Michael: Breaking the taboos

I am reserved when I share with others my experiences around entering and maneuvering a PhD program as a FGS. Sharing information about my family history and my experiences as a FGS within our group made me feel vulnerable. When I was growing up in rural farm settings of Iowa and Mississippi, these things were not talked about in my home. Neither of my parents completed high school, and my family emphasized hard work over education. At age 19, I remember telling my mother "This is not going to work for me," in an attempt to express and explain my desire to explore higher education at a community college. My approach was not well received. She defended the sharecropping farm work that she and my father learned as children and the work that supported my family for generations.

Sharing this with others, especially others in PhD programs, can be uncomfortable. I want to be seen as an academic. Sharing this with people who can relate is also normalizing for me. I have many identities, and like others in our group my FGS identity remains salient in addition to my identity as an academic. Even as a doctoral candidate, hopefully nearing the end of my PhD program, my identity as a FGS is on the surface. For example, the terminology and academic jargon used by some in academia can leave me feeling like an outsider. I am aware that, like all students, I am learning new information, but there are some words and concepts that many people just know as a result of growing up with parents, family members and other people who have a college education. There were times in meetings or classes when I felt like I needed a dictionary to participate. On those occasions I quickly asked myself if I wanted to search for more information using an application on my smart phone and risk being viewed as not paying attention, ask for clarification and risk appearing ignorant, or say nothing and risk not being able to follow the remainder of the discussion.

To counter those experiences, being a part of this group with other FGS is powerful—the concept of breaking taboos resonates with me around these experiences. Sharing these experiences with others helps me to see that this is normal for some of us in academia. I can actually say what I am thinking out loud and George or Michele will usually laugh. They laugh, not because they think I am being silly or stupid, but because they have either experienced the same thing or something similar.

Our group work insights

Entering the academy can be challenging for junior scholars who identify as FGS and who often enter academic programs with minimal knowledge on how to traverse the pathways of the academic elite (Gardner & Holley, 2011). The magic of the group process is such that it has provided a venue that is compelling and effective in bridging our success as FGS. In the reflection of our collective efforts to belong to the academy, we experienced three pivotal principles of group process: mutual aid, inclusion and respect, and breaking taboos.

As FGS, we skittishly came to realize that we all struggle with the imposter syndrome, a feeling that somehow we aren't smart enough to be in the academy. And the nagging fear that it is only a matter of time until we are exposed to our colleagues as frauds. We came to recognize that there is an institutionalized academic posturing. Uncertainty or doubt is frowned upon by the educated elite. Our own pursuit to prove our worthiness, to belong, often enslaves us to this ideology of self-sufficiency. Our reflection reminded us that this is in direct conflict with our understanding of mutual aid. We strive to dismantle the privileging of academic power used as a barrier to FGS. As social work practitioners and educators we experience this magic of vulnerability with our clients and students and we reaffirm our commitment to mutual aid and its power to bridge future FGS success.

We value inclusion and respect as a group process. Celebrating dimensions of differences unveils voices, beliefs, and experiences. During our revealing of who we are as individuals, we found an understanding of our similarities. In a climate of safety we were able to unpack the sting of "otherness." We found laughter in sharing our coping strategies and healing in revealing the often shadowed pain. Our collection of survival stories became a source of healing and support for one another in negotiating unique academic challenges, normalization of our feelings of otherness around academic privileging, and a reaffirmation of our value to the academy as FGS. Self and group reflections proved to be a potent process for recognizing the diversity of our group and for creating self-awareness.

Telling our stories and hearing about each other's experiences served as a means to use the power of our group to break the taboos that accompany the identity of FGS. In bringing our full selves from the shadows, we claim a wholeness. We acknowledge the value our FGS status brings to the academy. No longer a taboo our FGS status is, rightfully, a valued professional strength.

We share these narratives as a glimpse into our lives as FGS and illustrate the bonding factors that created our group. Our social group work exerted "extraordinary effectiveness in contradicting feelings of powerlessness and internalized self-hatred" (Drumm, 2006, p. 28). We share our stories in an effort to recognize our own transition into the educated elite and as a reminder of the educational journey of future FGS. We are committed to using our positions as social work practitioners, educators, and researchers to welcome more FGS into the academy.

References

Drumm, K. (2006). The essential power of group work. *Social Work with Groups, 29*(2/3), 17–31. doi:10.1300/J009v29n02_02

Gardner, S. K., & Holley, K. A. (2011). "Those invisible barriers are real": The progression of first-generation students through doctoral education. *Equity & Excellence in Education, 44*(1), 77–92. doi:10.1080/10665684.2011.529791

Malekoff, A. (2001). The power of group work with kids: A practitioner's reflection on strengths-based practice. *Families in Society, 82*(3), 243–249. doi:10.1606/1044-3894.197

The Village: Still Alive and Necessary

Samuel R. Benbow

A few months ago my sisters and I helped clean out our mother's garage, which stored a lifetime of memories and dormant feelings that were awakened as we worked our way through the many boxes, trying to decide what to keep and what to discard. I came across a button that had a Black Power raised fist draped in black, red, and green colors with the words, "It take a village to raise a child" inscribed. I took the button and put it in my pocket to show my daughters (ages 12 and 18) and share a few lessons. As I share my village experience that took place in Southwest Philadelphia, I ask that you consider getting in touch with your own village experience to become aware of its impact on you.

I was the youngest, and only male, of four poverty-stricken children raised in the late 1960s by a single parent mother, in the inner city of West Philadelphia better known as "the Bottom." Some of the significant events of this time period were the Vietnam War, Civil Rights Movement, Black Power Movement, the televised assassination of President John F. Kennedy, and, most importantly in my African American community, the assassination of Reverend Dr. Martin Luther King Jr. These events generated civil unrest and the oppression of many impoverished African American communities across the nation by law enforcement personnel.

The result of all this in my community was increased unemployment, poverty, single-parent homes, high school dropout rates, gang violence, and juvenile delinquency. I vividly recall several community leaders and activists giving speeches in front of the grocery stores and laundromats, handing out pamphlets and repeatedly calling out one of the prominent catch phrases of that era, "It takes a village to raise a child."

A young teenager I observed clothing, television commercials, and radio programs often using some version of the "It takes a village to raise a child" theme. I traced the roots of the catchphrase to an old African proverb in which members of a particular tribe believed in an inherent responsibility of and to all tribe members to teach, nurture, and when necessary, correct all children of the tribe with no consideration to biological affiliation or political connection. I wondered where my village in West Philadelphia was. Who were my elders? How did my elders help raise me? More importantly, am I now an elder? And, if so what does that mean?

Up until I was age 10 my village in West Philadelphia consisted of a four-block radius that was slowly being overtaken by colleges such as Drexel University and the University of Pennsylvania. Within my four blocks, the vast majority of those in power were a different color than me and included store owners, teachers, police officers, landlords, free clinic employees, and politicians. As we walked outside of the four blocks, houses looked different, streets were clean, there were no heroin clinics and only one or two fast food corner stores. In place of the local stores that catered primarily to food stamp recipients to buy a cheese steak or Italian hoagies, there were health food stores selling wheats, grains, oats, nuts and a wide variety of fresh fruits and vegetables.

When I turned 11 my family moved to Southwest Philadelphia for a better quality of living. My village more than doubled in size, expanding to a 10-block radius with all of the same resources, limitations, power structures, and opportunities. Being a little older afforded me the opportunity to venture out and to actually see the village and ultimately identify my elders.

My elders consisted of Mrs. Blackwell (seventyish), Lou (fortyish), Mrs. Kaye (sixtyish), Mrs. Barbara (seventyish), and Mrs. Etta (sixtyish); who I affectionately named my "Fantastic Five." My "Fantastic Five" were all African American women with adult children. They were retired or stay-at-home mothers who lived on my block. They kept me busy with odd jobs such as running errands to the grocery store, cutting grass, shoveling snow, vacuuming, dusting, changing cat litter, and washing windows. Oddly enough, I was politely pressured, on a weekly basis, to share my grades, my interests for the future, what I was doing with my friends, how I was treating my older sisters, and what it meant to respect my mother. As far as I am aware, they never talked to each other about how to raise me, but as I look back they were instrumental in charting my future as a father, husband, brother, son, and mentor. I was the client and they were the group, working to help me to find different path than my sisters who all dropped out of high school and became involved in drug and alcohol use and abuse.

More than 30 years later, as I write this story, I still have my elders (though they are different now) whom I affectionately call my mentors, friends, and colleagues. They are extremely diverse with regards to gender, sexual orientation, socioeconomic status, age, profession, and educational accomplishments. Like my original "Fantastic Five," I have recently realized that I am a budding elder, not necessarily by age, but definitely by experience and knowledge. In my role as an academic advisor, college professor, community activist, and social worker, I have come across a number of men whom I have worked with in my various capacities to help nurture their lives. Today, my "Fantastic Five" includes Clint (49-year-old Veteran who graduated from college recently and is working as a social worker), Travis (22-year-old college student, currently in his final year and planning to attend graduate school in Ireland for Sports Management and hopefully work for the International Olympic Committee), Vic (23-year-old recent college graduate, who will be working toward his graduate degree in counseling this fall), Daniel (20-year-old trying to start college in the fall for the third time), and Barry (29-year-old who graduated from college six short years ago, and is scheduled to leave for the United States Marine Corps (USMC) boot camp toward the end of August).

My "Fantastic Five" all had unique life challenges. They came into my life in completely different ways and are all committed to more than themselves. They vary in age, race, ethnicity, socioeconomic level, education, life experiences, living circumstances, career interests, as well as the conditions within which they were raised. Regardless of those differences, we have formed a life-long mutual aid group. As an elder of the group, I unintentionally connected various members of the group with each other based on what was going on at that particular time in their lives. I realized a number of years ago that I didn't have to have all the answers and that the five individuals I was helping shared common interests and could be of support to one another and me. For example, when Barry was first contemplating enlisting in the Marine Corps, he reached out to me because I too served in the Marine Corps some 30 years ago. I connected Barry to Clint, who then reached out to a friend and a recruiter in the Corps. They met via face time several times over the past few months helping him prepare physically, emotionally, and spiritually for his life in the military (for him, his wife, and his child).

The "Fantastic Five" is a wonderful example of the benefit of a naturally formed mutual aid group in a social media--driven society. Location, access, and support are instantly available in a respectful and healthy manner. Tough love is given with no regard to softening the reality blow because our differences of age, race, ethnicity, social economic status, sexual orientation, and life experiences. We check in with each other for help, support, and reinforcement of our collective and individual sanity. We do not use Facebook or Twitter, just old fashioned e-mail and cell phones to communicate. We have become friends who support one another.

For example, in a recent conversation with Barry I shared that my family has been busy emotionally preparing for my oldest daughter's departure for college in a few short weeks. He knows that we are a very close family and that, though we are very excited, it's still very hard for our family. As I was fighting to hold back one or two tears, Barry shared his thoughts and feelings on such a sensitive topic. Without hesitation or concerned about my role or status in the group, he said, "You got this! How many of us did you help make it?" While we were talking, he started texting and I got quiet trying to gather my own thoughts before addressing the fact that he was texting while we were talking. Barry shared that, "Daniel has a cousin at my daughter's college and he is going to give her your number, so expect a call." In a world where privacy and confidentiality has served to dramatically increase lawsuits, my contact information was given without hesitation. Awesome!

As a budding elder I can see how the village/mutual aid group is continuing to help me grow, develop, and soar while I help the "Fantastic Five" do the same. My role as the "social worker/group facilitator" has been replaced with elder. We have made a commitment to take a "man" trip to Parris Island in Beaufort, South Carolina, for Barry's graduation in December. Although we will be heading to Parris Island from different parts of the United States, I believe that it is my responsibility as well as other elders in our society; to make sure all of our "group members" understand where they came from and encourage them to make the ultimate commitment of helping those who they mentor to succeed.

Our village members traversed a variety of social and emotional landscapes to guide direct and support each other, all the while respecting one another's differences. As Daniel is the newest member to our village, he's learned quickly that the other members are nonthreatening and have no hidden agendas. He trusts me, "the elder," and by extension he trusts all of our "village members."

In closing, our village code is simply to trust each other, provide support, and keep it real. As I have accepted my role as a budding elder, I ask you to reflect on your own professional and personal life to answer a few questions. "Are you an elder? Where is your village? Who are the members of your village? How are you helping your village to grow?"

As your seasons change, I hope that by sharing my experience navigating the natural mutual aid groups of my youth and later years—my "Fantastic Fives"—that you will consider the role you play, can play, in helping to make our neighborhoods and communities a better place to live, grow and learn, one group at a time.

Index

Note: Page numbers in *italic* type refer to figures
Page numbers followed by 'n' refer to notes